Parkour

Basic Parkour Strength and Movement

(The Complete Guide to Parkour and Freerunning for Beginners)

Denise Rivera

Published By **Jordan Levy**

Denise Rivera

All Rights Reserved

Parkour: Basic Parkour Strength and Movement (The Complete Guide to Parkour and Freerunning for Beginners)

ISBN   978-1-7780579-1-5

No part of this guidebook shall be reproduced in any form without permission in writing from the publisher except in the case of brief quotations embodied in critical articles or reviews.

Legal & Disclaimer

The information contained in this ebook is not designed to replace or take the place of any form of medicine or professional medical advice. The information in this ebook has been provided for educational & entertainment purposes only.

The information contained in this book has been compiled from sources deemed reliable, and it is accurate to the best of the Author's knowledge; however, the Author cannot guarantee its accuracy and validity and cannot be held liable for any errors or omissions. Changes are periodically made to this book. You must consult your doctor or get professional medical advice before using any of the suggested remedies, techniques, or information in this book.

Upon using the information contained in this book, you agree to hold harmless the

Author from and against any damages, costs, and expenses, including any legal fees potentially resulting from the application of any of the information provided by this guide. This disclaimer applies to any damages or injury caused by the use and application, whether directly or indirectly, of any advice or information presented, whether for breach of contract, tort, negligence, personal injury, criminal intent, or under any other cause of action.

You agree to accept all risks of using the information presented inside this book. You need to consult a professional medical practitioner in order to ensure you are both able and healthy enough to participate in this program.

TABLE OF CONTENTS

INTRODUCTION 1

CHAPTER 1. WHAT EXACTLY IS PARKOUR? 4

CHAPTER 2: BACKGROUND OF PARKOUR AND FREERUNNING 23

CHAPTER 3: TIPS TO STAY RELIABLE AND SAFE 34

CHAPTER 4: UNDERSTANDING YOUR BODY 47

CHAPTER 5: UNDERSTANDING THE CONCEPTS OF TRAINING 53

CHAPTER 6: RUNNING AND BALANCING 61

CHAPTER 7: JUMPING AND LANDING 64

CHAPTER 8: THE VAULTS 72

CHAPTER 9: CLIMBING 76

CHAPTER 10: THE SWINGING AND HANGING 80

CHAPTER 11: DEFINE FREE RUNNING 86

CHAPTER 12: THE STORY OF FREE RUNNING 88

CHAPTER 13: THE PHILOSOPHY OF FREE RUNNING 93

CHAPTER 14: FREE-RUN MOVEMENTS 97

CHAPTER 15: THE RISKS OF FREE RUNNING 99

CHAPTER 16: FREE RUNNING EQUIPMENT 103

CHAPTER 17: THE DEVELOPMENT OF FREE RUNNING 105

CHAPTER 18: FUTURE OF FREE RUNNING 109

CHAPTER 19: DEFINE PARKOUR AND FREERUNNING 111

CHAPTER 20: AMERICAN NINJA WARRIOR COMPETITION 115

CHAPTER 21: THE APPLICATION PROCESS 118

CHAPTER 22: THE AMERICAN NINJA WORKOUT 122

CHAPTER 23: SURVIVING THE TOUGHEST OBSTACLES ... 145

CHAPTER 24: NINJA NUTRITION 154

CHAPTER 25: FINDING THE JOB 173

CONCLUSION 184

Introduction

This book is written intended for those who are looking to learn the basics of Free Running and are not in a position to know where to start or what data to rely on. This book was written in response to the growing demand from people who want to learn the basics of Free Running and why it is the trend that is coming. The Internet contains a wealth of misinformation and articles regarding Free Running that confuse the individuals who are curious about this new trend and may be looking to test it for themselves.

This book I'm going to provide you with an uncomplicated guide to everything you need to learn about Free-Rounding/Parkour. In addition, we will look at the background of Free Running and Parkour, the present state of the game, and the equipment required to ensure that you will be able to comprehend the vital facts before trying it on your own. It doesn't matter if you're planning on trying it out or would like to know more about the reasons why this sport is gaining popularity It is crucial to be aware of the benefits and potential risks.

I would suggest taking notes when you are reading this book. It will allow you to are getting the most value from the content. I hope that you feel like you bought something that's worth the money and that's why you are able to go through the notes in the book after having completed reading it. Notes will allow you identify exactly what you'll need to be able to recall and, by writing things down it will help you to recall details.

Remember that this book was compiled by conducting research, my personal experiences, and the experiences of other people, so you are free to ask questions about the information you've learned inside this text. I suggest that you do your own research into those topics you'd like to learn more about. The more you know about Free Running/Parkour, the better informed your decision-making process is in regards to taking a spin or providing tips to other people.

Chapter 1. What exactly is Parkour?

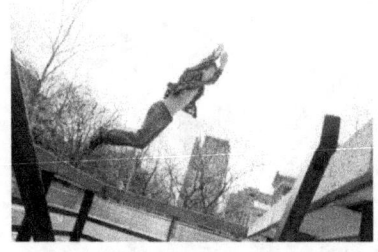

Parkour is about moving around your surroundings quickly and effortlessly. Parkour practitioners, typically referred to as traceuers (from the French meaning to trace) are able to jump, climb and jump over obstacles along their way. Their aim is to move from point A to B as quickly as they can.

The story of parkour's history is quite interesting. It was developed in France and is rooted in the military strategies for escape and evasion as well as the 19th century's physical culture. Actually, the term "parkour" is derived from the French expression "parcours du combattant" the obstacle course-based training method that was used in soldiers in the French military. While we may think of parkour as an enjoyable form of recreation the fact is that it was designed as a tactic skill as a way to improve the physical fitness of soldiers.

What is the difference between Parkour and Freerunning

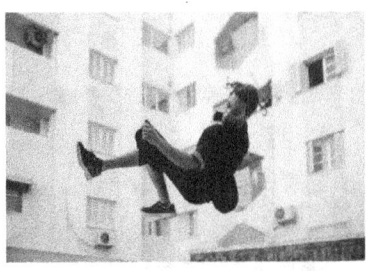

Parkour and freerunning are utilized in a variety of ways. Although they have a lot in common, they have one minor difference.

Parkour is about simply moving through your surroundings efficiently with swings, jumps, and vaults. You don't need flips, wall spins and other Acrobatics. Freerunning is efficient and much less of an issue and you can incorporate these types of cool-looking acrobatics in addition.

When you're viewing YouTube video clips of individuals performing flips and spins on walls, they're doing freerunning. If they're simply jumping and soaring over urban obstacles with no the ability to perform acrobatics then they're parkour.

Why do you want to practice parkour?

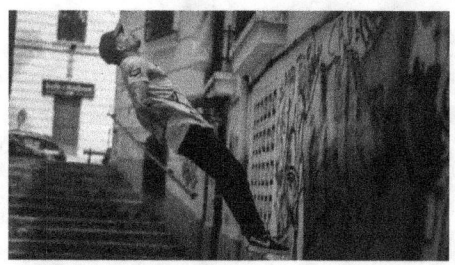

It's enjoyable! It is a sport where you consider the world around you as the size of a playground. It's enjoyable to come up with new ways to navigate your surroundings, and do you really think you're escaping from zombies, ninjas, or even ninja assassi. It awakens the child in you who has been secluded for a long time and wants to play around, explore the world without limit and just play.

Parkour is an excellent way to exercise. Running, jumping, climbing, swinging. Parkour is a full body workout that simultaneously increases your coordination and body awareness.

Parkour is a test. Parkour requires you to challenge yourself both mentally and physically. In the beginning, you may not be able to perform certain movements, but over time, you'll develop the coordination and strength you require to master them. There will be obstacles you believe you'll never overcome, but once you really look within you'll discover that you're pushing your body to the limits of the limits you thought were its limits. In short, it helps activate the primordial human instinct within each of us to take on an adventure. When you conquer these obstacles, you'll build confidence in yourself, which can be carried over to different areas that you live.

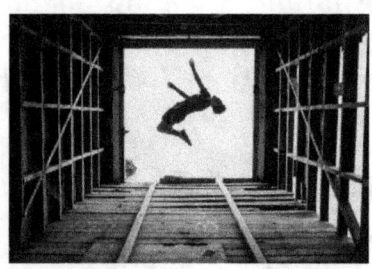

Parkour is a fantastic method to make new friends. Parkour is a game that can be played in a group. It is usually played in groups and the community of parkour is extremely supportive and friendly. It's not a sport of competition; instead, the aim is having a fun time and assist each other in improving.

Parkour could you save your life. We're huge supporters of the belief that everyone is capable of saving his own life if the need arises. Parkour provides the ability and physical fitness to accomplish this. We talk about zombies and needing to escape or escape urban environments however what happens do you do if your life is dependent on being capable of running, jumping and leap over obstacles? Are you able to accomplish it? Parkour can help. It's especially useful when you need to leap from roof to roof.

Parkour helps you be more imaginative. Parkour demands you think about your surroundings in a creative way. Instead of interfacing and moving across the globe as an urban planner or architect wanted you to do, you simply perform it in the way you like. Stairs? We don't need no stinkin' stairs! Do you would like me to utilize this tiny bridge for pedestrians? I'll simply jump over this gap and slide under this rail. Every wall, fence, or gap is an opportunity to play with some new moves. This type of playfulness and creative thinking can spread into other aspects that you live in, assisting you come up with creative solutions to issues in your work environment or relationships.

How to Begin With Parkour

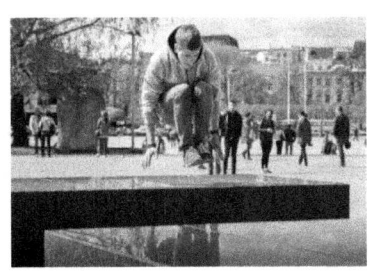

Find a group of parkour. The most effective way to begin in the sport of parkour is to locate a local club and go to an event like a jam. The community of parkour players are extremely welcoming and supportive of each other. You'll gain insights from people who've been practicing for some time, and also have someone watching the most difficult moves. Also, in the event that you fall badly and fall, there's someone who will bring them to hospital. The majority of cities offer parkour meetings; you will locate them on Meetup.com and on the american Parkour forums.

Another way for starting would be joining a parkour-based gym such as that of the Tempest Freerunning Academy if you're fortunate enough to have one located in your region. These kinds of gyms are relatively new, and there's not any available currently, however more are likely to pop in the coming decades as parkour continues to increase in popularity.

Take precautions. Do not take risks that aren't necessary. The goal is simply to enjoy a great experience and to push your self to the edge of your comfortable zone, not causing injury to yourself. The first thing to ask before performing any exercise should be "How do I accomplish this without hurting me?" Make sure to train in a group or with an instructor to identify you during difficult movements and seek assistance when needed. Before every training session, make sure to check the surroundings for potential dangers, such as broken glass, for instance. So, don't make a mistake.

Be patient. Know your limits. Even if others are performing insane aerials and flips from massive structures, doesn't mean that you must. Be careful not to try too much in too short a time. It'll take a while before your body can adjust to the demands of the physical nature of parkour. Don't attempt more complex moves until you've perfected the fundamentals. In a similar vein Don't be so confident about your ability that you don't consider every move with a serious. Pride can lead to fall and in parkour, the fall could be very damaging.

Be respectful of private property. Make sure you do parkour only in public spaces such as parks and plazas for cities. Be sure to stay clear of times that have large pedestrians. If someone asks you to leave, you should politely reply, "Sure thing!" If you are confronted by the police Be courteous, be prepared to explain your actions, and abide by requests to go somewhere and not elsewhere. Parkour is an upcoming and unheard of game in U.S. Any thing you could do to help give Parkour a positive name can help make it more popular.

Basic Parkour Movements

Balancing

Balancing is an essential ability to master in parkour. It is common to walk and jumping onto small spaces like rails and walls edges. It is important to build the strength and coordination so that you don't fall into the ground. Balance by walking or standing on rails. You might want to consider slacklining as a way to improve your balance.

Running

To successfully avoid zombies and other dangerous pursuing creatures in a city environment you must run. Parkour running requires fast and explosive sprinting, as well as endurance. The practice of parkour on a regular basis can prepare you for the endurance required for running, but you should consider adding 5K and windprints to increase speed.

Jumping and dropping

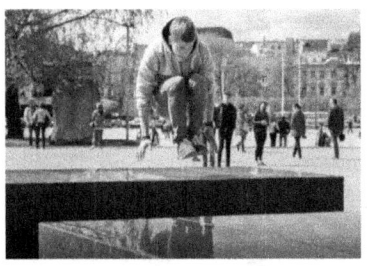

Jumping is an integral part in parkour. Jumps are a great way to overcome the differences in height and to go across gaps and jump over obstacles..

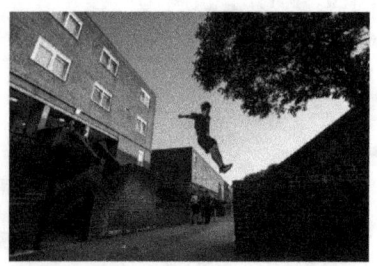

Precision jumping

Precision jumps permit you to be able to land on tiny places, like the small area on the wall's top or perhaps some stepping stones within the water body. Precision jumps require focus in balance, balance, and awareness of your own limitations.

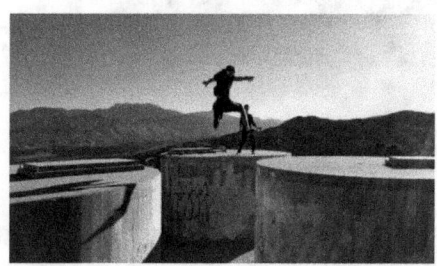

Tic-Tac

Tic-tacs can be described as an amalgamation of a wall climb and the jump. This allows you to climb to heights that are higher than what you can with a leap. You've probably seen them in films about martial arts or American Ninja Warrior. It's when a person walks toward a wall from an angle, then places one foot against the wall then pushes away from the wall using that foot to leap into a higher height. Tic-tacs typically are utilized in conjunction with another move.

Drop

A drop is a leap from a high to lower level. If you're just beginning out in parkour, be careful not to drop from heights that are higher than the head level. It is important to learn how to land (see further below) and prepare your body for the pressure that comes with being able to drop from heights.

Landing

Being able to land safely and effectively after dropping or jumping is a crucial skill to master for freerunning and parkour. Achieving a good landing will allow you to instantly move on to the next obstacle and, most importantly it means you don't have to visit the hospital emergency rooms.

The way you make your landing depends on several elements, including: 1)) the distance you'll be landing from, 2.) the distance you leap three) the surface you'll land on, and four) the previous jump you made.

Two-foot landing

Two-foot landings are better than one-foot landings in lessening the stress your body feels upon landing. If you are able make it to landing in two steps. If you do make it to the ground, you should need that your initial contact the heels with shoulder width apart with knees positioned over the tips of your toes.

The goal is to get down in as "softly" as you can. To ensure a soft landing make sure to bend your knees as you land , but be sure that they do not bend more than 90 °. If you're dropping or jumping from a very high height or landing with lots or forward speed, you should let your body sink toward your legs and put your hands on the ground so that your arms are able to absorb the force. The hands being placed on the ground will also put you in a good position to rise up and race towards your next hurdle. This kind of landing requires time, so practice from lower levels prior to moving onto the next level.

Rolling

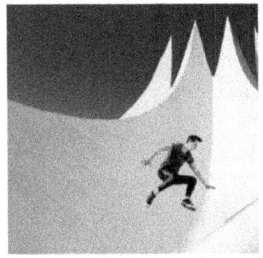

Rolling is a crucial landing skill that you should master in order to stay safe from injuries. After landing, rolling distributes the impact force across different parts of your body to reduce the chance of injuries. You'll usually want to go into a roll immediately after landing when you're falling from high heights or leaping in a horizontal direction with a high forward speed. If done correctly, a roll can let you fall and then bounce right back up without a scratch on your skin.

You're supposed to roll on your shoulder in a diagonal direction across your back, so that you're moving between one hip and the other hip. Put your head down under your armpit while you move in the circle. Focus on circling your body and forming yourself into the shape of a ball. Stay in a tight position while your weight pulls you through the roll. Keep the knees straight and keep your body weight in the lowest position when you climb to your feet.

Vaulting

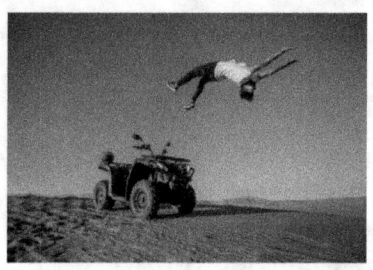

When you're running, you'll come across obstacles that are just too high for you to leap over. This is where vaulting comes in. Vaulting involves placing your hands on a object to aid in clearing it. There are a variety of vaults that you can choose from in accordance with your obstacle remove and your personal preferences. Brian Orosco from Tempest Freerunning Academy presented us with five typical vaults that are used in freerunning and parkour. They are shown in the video below. I've also added links to a variety of parksour websites that provide steps-by-step instructions for the vaults too.

The Step (safety) vault. The step vault is the simplest vault to construct and provides the foundation for the other vaults. It is usually done when you are moving towards an obstacle in a slow manner.

Speed vault. Like the name implies the speed vault is done while you are running at full speed.

Lazy Vault. This is a great vault for when you are approaching the obstacle from an angle. It's likely that you've done this type of vault with no idea about it was possible when you were when you were a child. When your body is swaying over the obstacle with no feet touching the ground and you only have one hand placed on the obstacle, you're performing the speed vault.

Kong Vault. Kong vaults can make you appear like you're jumping over police vehicles as Caesar from Rise of the Planet of the Apes. This is a highly advanced vaulting technique. Make sure that you've gained some knowledge in parkouring.

Dash Vault. Dash vault works sort of similar to Kong vault. Kong vault, with the exception that it is a leap first, instead of head first.

Climbing

Stairs are meant for people who are chumps. Sometimes it's better to choose an easy route to reach the next niveau. This is where climbing comes in. Begin slowly with climbing at first when you're beginning with parkour. There aren't any safety harnesses, and the chance of falling from a high point could land you hospitalized or be six feet below. The general rule for doing parkour climbing is "don't climb any higher than you are able to leap down." In addition to the basic "ladder" type climbingtechniques, there's different climbing techniques that you should be conscious of.

Wall run

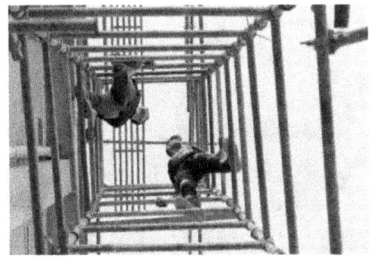

Wall runs permit you to climb up a very tall wall and do it very quickly. Wall runs are an incredibly complex move. It's one of the most prominent obstacles that is featured on American Ninja Warrior, but it's one that many participants have difficulty with. In order to successfully complete wall runs, you need to jump, run to, climb, and hang all in one smooth movement - which isn't as easy as it seems.

Cat leaps

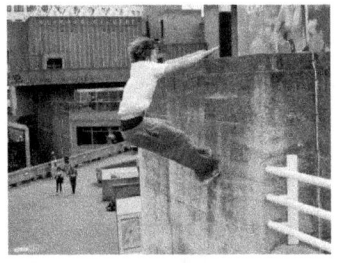

A cat jump is mix of the two. The cat leap is used in situations where you must span an opening, but the landing area is too high to be able to stand on your feet. Therefore, you must hang on to your hands as you make your way to the other end. When you're hanging from an edge on the wall or building then pull yourself up to safe by bringing your knees towards your chest, and then pressing your toes against the wall. Lift your legs by your toes while pulling your body upwards with your hands simultaneously. Make sure to push your legs as they'll possess the strength and strength over your arms. Once your shoulders are clear of the edge of the ledge, make sure that your palms are level against the top of the ledge. Straighten your arms and then push your body upwards. Lean forward to ensure that you're center of gravity lies on your side of safety, so that you're not prone to fall should you fall off balance.

Swinging

The swinging of trees or a tree is often used in parkour. There are many traceurs who make use of swings to traverse an obstacle when there's gap between the rail and the surface.

Apart from the underbar swing as a basic You can also be a bit more sophisticated with the spiral swing underbar. In essence, you grip the bar in a manner that makes you spin when you swing beneath the bar. This is pretty cool.

Chapter 2: Background of Parkour and Freerunning

Freerunning and parkour are both relatively young sports that have evolved out of a mere ideology in the last 200 years. Both of these sports were developed in France. David Belle is known to be the founder of parkour as well as Sebastian Foucan is considered to be the father of freerunning.

This chapter I'll present the numerous factors that have allowed the two art forms to develop to what they are in the present. This chapter starts with the contributions of the 20th century by Georges Hebert.

Methode Naturelle

The philosophical basis of parkour is the methode naturel (natural method) which was a method of training that was developed in the 20th century by French navy official Georges Hebert in the 20th century. In honor of its founder this method, it is often known as the Hebertisme.

Georges Hebert was a firm fan of physical fitness. He believed that everyone should engage in daily physical exercise. This was because he believed that physically fit and athletic individuals could help their communities, in particular in regards to development and protection. Hebert's source of inspiration is the individuals he visited in his travels through

Africa. He noticed that, while the indigenous people were close to the natural world but their bodies were strong and agile. They also had a strong and durable physique.

In 1902, a volcano eruption destroyed in the French island Martinique. In the time that Hebert was stationed on Martinique He was able organize the evacuation in a safe manner of nearly 700 residents of Martinique. His views were strengthened by this. physical fitness was essential in addition to valor and charity in order for people to be able to assist the community.

This is why he decided to concentrate on fitness training after the return trip to France. At Reims, at the University of Reims, Hebert was the leader of a strict fitness program that consisted of lifting, running as well as jumping in natural settings. The diverse training plans were developed to train students to to endure and excel in any natural terrain, no matter what the conditions.

The main concern was not contests, but Hebert believed that it distracted students from the essence of his curriculum. To further reinforce his belief in natural method, Hebert developed an obstacle course that mimicked natural situations. He was among the first to develop this outside of the military.

The methods of training used by Hebert greatly affected the military training that was provided by The French government. Soldiers have adapted Hebert's techniques to operate in the unforgiving terrain of Vietnam during the Vietnam War.

Hebert utilized the term "roue» to describe the instruction of his courses that was similar to the military's use of the term"roue of combattant (which literally refers to an the assault-course). The current use of parkour is considered to be the natural application of the method in urban or industrial environments which are becoming more prevalent as opposed to natural landscapes. The parkour players are required to comprehend the methods of training used by Hebert to be more physically and mentally able to navigate through the various situations.

Natural Gymnastics

The framework for education in the West was fundamentally altered from the latter half of 19th century and the beginning of the 20th century. In contrast to treating pupils as objects through whom teachers impart knowledge, the advent of the educational progressivism revolutionized the way in which students were treated as individuals, each possessing the capacity to develop and grow.

Before this it was viewed as a thorough ability to master a set of movements. It was a far cry from its origins that required individuals to grow as an individual.

In the wake of educational progressivism In the wake of educational progressivism, two Austrians with the names of Karl Gaulhofer and Margarete Streicher came up with the idea that natural gymnastics was a good idea. Instead of requiring students to do certain movements natural gymnastics encouraged creative
movements. Additionally, even the most ineffective moves in gymnastics can be

used as learning opportunities to find rapid and efficient methods of moving.

This groundbreaking gymnastics training rapidly spread to nearby Germany, France, and even across the world in the west. This was the reason that has inspired Raymond Belle and his son, David, the latter who would eventually develop parkour as an independent art form.

Raymond as well as David Belle

It is believed that the Frenchman Raymond Belle was born in the present day Vietnam in Vietnam, where he soon became abandoned. At the age of 12 years old, his family was already preparing him to join the French army. The majority of his youth was focused on physical fitness and also practicing the most efficient and effective escape techniques to survive the harsh conditions of Vietnam.

When he was a young adult, Raymond Belle moved to France in the year 2000, where he was an employee of the Paris Fire Brigade. The training and experience he gained from early childhood was passed through to his two sons, Jean-Francois as well as David.

David Belle was born in 1973 in the countryside of Fecamp and was nurtured in the home of his grandpa. As a young man, David Belle preferred to practice gymnastics in nature. This was due to his father's advice on the value of knowing about natural terrain. He was always trying to come up with methods to conquer obstacles in imagined situations where his bravery and ability could be put to the test.

David Belle and his family relocated to the city of industrial of Lisses when he was just 15 years old. Being unable to access fields and forests, Belle practiced his moves in urban areas. His performances drawn a lot of other youngsters.

One of the best friends Belle has made is Sebastian Foucan. Sebastian and Belle were always chasing each other around the modern city of Lisses. But as the boys grew older they changed their way of running around the city. The two boys became more adept at maneuvering around obstacles. They described the game they invented the art of deplacement (the art of Displacement).

The group comprised of Belle, Foucan, and many others developed the methods that are part of The Art of Displacement. The group gained more attention, however after David's brother Jean-Francois, who was a friend of his, presented a clip showing David and his companions to an audience on a French television show. After receiving a lot of media coverage, David Belle and his friends joined forces to form their group Yamakasi.

"The Art of Displacement

When the Yamakasi members Yamakasi created The Art of Displacement, they believed that it was similar to George Hebert's philosophies. They devised the techniques to create the Art of Displacement with some understanding of the philosophy of Hebert.

Yamakasi became a well-known group within a couple of years. Its name is the Art of Displacement developed certain movements that drew inspiration from different disciplines and sports. Although Yamakasi is considered to be the very first parkour and freerunning group, the two names aren't in use yet. In the end, Belle and Foucan each quit the group in order to further develop the Art by utilizing techniques that they wanted to pursue. Even though they left however, the group Yamakasi continues to exist to the present.

Parkour

In the time that David Belle and Sebastian Foucan quit Yamakasi the group, they were forced to leave because of the different methods used by the group. They took with them The Art of Displacement. This Art of Displacement, however was gradually modified to meet the standards set by or Belle and Foucan.

In the case of David Belle, speculations say that he was looking to honor his father. While he was not referring to the art in the name of Art of Displacement, he changed it's name to parkour (from George Hebert's route). Belle reduced the various aspects of parkour to what was his perception of it when he was growing up. Parkour was a focus on efficient movement and escape strategies that were a reflection of the experiences of his father when he was a young soldier in his father's French army.

As the world gained access to access to television, many were fascinated by The Art of Displacement as well as the things Belle and Foucan could offer. But, despite its popularity, David Belle did not think about developing parkour any further. Instead, he pursued a degree in English and then became an actor. He has been in a variety of films and been stunt coordinator for many of Hollywood's most popular films.

Freerunning

Sebastian Foucan deviated from David Belle's strategy of efficient movement and created freerunning. Freerunning, unlike parkour, isn't founded on ideology to make it more adaptable to various situations.

The growing popularity of freerunning and parkour it sparked heated debates regarding which features belong to each. Many of the practitioners have begun to incorporate the acrobatics of their sport, which didn't meet the definition of parkour of effectiveness and freedom. This is why other innovative and acrobatic actions in urban settings are categorized as freerunning. In the present, both freerunning and parkour are regarded as distinct disciplines.

Chapter 3: Tips to Stay Reliable and Safe

Because freerunning and parkour are sports that require active participation anyone who wants to participate in either of them must be conscious of the essential precautions. Being injured is a typical consequence of engaging in freerunning or parkour. You need to learn to ensure that your actions and stunts are safe and safe.

Help received from Belle and Foucan

Even though David Belle and Sebastian Foucan might not have been able to agree on what the proper moves should be for Art of Displacement, both were adamant about certain specific values that ensure the security and integrity of the performer whenever he does tricks in freerunning or parkour.

To David Belle, free movement is not a given. Parkour although beautiful and fluid, is grounded in the concept of the best way to move through the city in a certain way. To become proficient in parkour you should not just work on endurance, speed, and strength, but also be aware of your body, and be confident in your in control and an capability to adapt to any circumstance.

David Belle also wants parkour athletes to be modest determination, willpower and endurance. In the eyes of Belle all parkour enthusiasts must be aware of his limitations. While this shouldn't stop the ability of a person to do certain movements however, it should not hinder him from working hard to eventually get competent enough to master the art of parkour.

Sebastian Foucan agrees to some degree that the runner should become conscious of his body and its limitations. However, the philosophy of Foucan in freerunning is influenced by eastern beliefs and practices. Foucan created the concept of "following your own path" to ensure that the unified body, spirit , and the surrounding can seamlessly and harmoniously interconnect.

Foucan has provided 12 values that freerunners should adhere to.

1. Be sure to follow your path. You are your own worst enemy However, you're the body you are. Follow the exercises

that you feel comfortable with, however, you should not jump into any movements that you might like, but that aren't within your abilities. Try freerunning or parkour at an amount that feels suitable.

2. It is important to practice regularly. No one is an expert in a short time. Training allows you to comprehend the art in a deeper way as well as to understand what limitations, and opportunities your body has to face.

3. Respect each other. Every person is unique. You can't dictate your way of doing things against others. You should let them choose their own way of life. In the absence of that, you cannot provide them with some advice. Be sure to treat your fellows with respect, just as you treat yourself.

4. Be an inspiration to other runners. Freerunning doesn't take its own sport seriously. Therefore, freerunners should be more interested in advancing the art of running through continuous practice and creating an inclusive community.

5. Keep positive and live in positive surroundings. In Foucan's eastern-influenced philosophy, could interfere with one's relationship with his self, the mind, and the environment. To be an ethical freerunner, or an expert in parkour one must be able to set the right intentions to stop yourself from engaging in something that could be harmful or dangerous.

6. Respect your surroundings. Freerunning is a form of movement within a urban setting. You should not or should not destroy the surroundings in the course of executing or practicing the specific movement. Foucan would like you to be part of the world, and not place the environment below you as an instrument.

7. Discover other disciplines. Because freerunning is a sport that is based on imagination, do not feel limited by the current rules that can limit your expression. If you're not destructive, you could begin by trying other sports and maybe even take what you have learned into freerunning. Freerunning isn't the only sport that is suitable for everyone.

8. Don't take it too seriously. As an exercise, it's also an art, and an everyday way of life. It doesn't expect anything from you except your enthusiasm and commitment. There's no reason for you to be too concerned about it since it isn't your whole life.

9. Be present in the moment instead of worrying about the future. If you choose to live your method, the most important thing is to ensure that, at any point in time, you're capable of enjoying and expressing your personality. Freerunning can be considered an art form, however, it's not a sport. It is not necessary to be the most impressive exhibitor to be recognized as freerunner. Take advantage of the experience and learn from every chance.

10. The only proper thing to do is to learn from your mistakes. As a result of the previous idea, freerunning is incredibly personal to you. Remember that the performance of freerunning depend on the way you are interacting with your surroundings. So that you take care of your surroundings, you are allowed to experiment with your actions.

11. Freerunning is not just restricted to a few, it is for those who are passionate about and who want to keep active. If you want to be a professional freerunner, be aware that anyone can participate in the sport. The complete refusal of interested persons from taking part for any reason will not be able to meet the sense of camaraderie that is expected from activities like freerunning or parkour.

12. Concentrate on your efforts in a positive method: a way to become better. The only thing you compete with is yourself and you have to keep in mind to enjoy yourself. When you engage in sports like freerunning and parkour You must realize that the primary reason for engaging is that it's enjoyable to you. If you believe this, you concentrate on improving your performance instead of being competitive or showing off. These do not fit the freerunning or parkour philosophies. parkour.

General safety tips

Parkour-related or freerunning events, particularly those that are viewed by the masses online are often extremely dangerous or even unwise. This is due to the security measures of the shows are usually removed from the video in order to boost the popularity of the video.

The general public has an inaccurate impression that freerunning and parkour are highly risky sports. However, this may be the case but it doesn't necessarily be the case. People should be aware that the performers in these videos are professionals as well as that security precautions had been taken prior to the production for the film.

The most common mistake novices do when they are practicing freerunning or parkour is that they try it by themselves. In the beginning you're at most risk of getting injured and property damages. It is best to join small groups or having a person who can assist you if an unexpected event occur. For those who are completely new to the field It is best to sign up for classes instead of taking a class in the event that you are unable to find a friend or a secure space to learn in.

But, it's not enough that you are practicing with the company. It is essential to ensure that you're in good company. Always be aware of your boundaries. Do not succumb to peer pressure to do something that you think is beyond your abilities. You're taking unneeded risks that could easily be avoided if you weren't pushed to perform the task.

A second thing to consider is to begin by doing exercises close to the ground. Anyone who was enthralled by the viral videos of parkour may feel the need to immediately try their hand at tall buildings or in elevated areas like bridges. It isn't safe and should be put off taking on this type of activity until you've at least two years of professional experience.

In the same way that you should be capable of respecting your surroundings by being mindful not to damage the property of private or public and also be conscious of your personal body. You are the only person who knows if you're suffering from an injury or illness. Always keep a first-aid kit with you whenever you train.

When you notice something that isn't right in your body, get it checked as quickly as you can. Don't force yourself into continuing your training. This is among essential safety guidelines for novices.

Training facilities

Because both parkour and freerunning can be done in urban environments It is normal to exercise outdoors. However it is true that not all outdoor areas are suitable for training. While scouting possible training sites, be sure to inspect the area and take note of any issues with structural strength (such as flooring or walls that are weak) and any security hazards (such as rough surfaces or sharp debris).

Be aware of the surfaces that are rusty, such as the roof or scaffolding. If you suffer a cut from these areas, you may be diagnosed with tetanus and necessitate you visiting your doctor right away. Tetanus, an illness brought on through the bacteria Clostridium Tetani, is thought to cause muscle spasms that are uncontrollable and lockjaw.

You must also be aware of the weather or climate. As traceurs are attracted by areas that are affected by snow or rain due to the innovative escape strategies they may come up with, beginners should stay away from slippery and wet surfaces at all times. It is advised to practice in protected areas when the season is one that brings snow or rain.

A few basic movements such as freerunning or parkour however, need to be learned by constant training. This is why it could be extremely beneficial to practice indoors , such as in gyms where floor padding or foam can be found.

When you train on your own, especially when you are trying new moves that you've learned through others or via videos It is recommended to do it under an experienced instructor. If supervision isn't available you can perform the exercises in an inflatable pit or an enormous area of water like an outdoor pool. They can greatly reduce the force from the falls, decreasing the risk of injury.

Training apparel is essential.

If you are choosing the appropriate clothing to train in, the most important needs are support and comfort to allow for freedom of movement.

There isn't any gear to be worn on the head. A beanie can prove useful in very cold conditions. It is not recommended to wear cap-styles that are fitted or other kinds of caps. The beanie is lightweight and has a non-obtrusive design that can support your movements particularly during rolls.

To wear clothes that you wear, a wide selection of clothes is recommended. T-shirts, sweatshirts, as well as long-sleeved tees are suitable in accordance with the weather and the way you feel at ease. Long-sleeved clothing can shield your skin from cuts or grazes during practice, and even decrease the chance of infection from any cuts. For the pants sweatpants are the standard attire. In contrast to other sports, there's no need to purchase special clothes.

In terms of shoes the only thing you require is a pair that has a great grip. The shoes you choose to wear must be near your foot so that you can be able to execute precise leaps and moves. You can pick any kind of sole you're comfortable with. There are specific shoes for freerunning and parkour and freerunning, which are recommended to buy if your local shop offers them.

If not, I would not suggest you buy expensive shoes for running or sports as they are likely to wear out every time you exercise. Shoes with inserts also help you more when you drop from higher elevations.

Cycling gloves can be helpful particularly for dealing with rough surfaces. The absence of a covering for your fingers can provide greater grip. Shin guards can also shield against scrapes if you fall. However, many traceurs as well as freerunners are against this , as well as other types devices for protection, saying that they are impeded in their movement. Although this could be the case but as a newbie you must put your safety above the quality of your movement.

The other items you need to train with include water, a first-aid kit, extra clothing, and towels. Put all these items in your sports bag so that you don't need to be burdened with them.

Chapter 4: Understanding Your Body

Before I can guide you through proper training methods You must first be aware of your body. Understanding anatomy and physiology will allow you to get greater results in a shorter time and also avoid potential injuries. In this article I will first discuss the theories behind nutrition, and then present the human muscles of the skeletal system.

Energy and the body

Before we talk about the bones we depend on for our actions, we should first be aware of where and how they obtain their energy at all. As a potential freerunner or traceur is basically an athlete. In this regard, you should be aware of the appropriate nutrition and which foods to consume more or stay clear of.

Due to the hefty nature of freerunning and parkour the athletes need more energy than people of average age. Living things are powered by the food they consume. Energy is measured by means of heat. The measurement is known as the Calorie (also called

Kilocalorie or 1000 calories, with a tiny "C").

In essence, the greater your activity, the hotter your body will become. This is due to the fact that you are taking in a lot of calories to make energy. If you're not active the body becomes chilled and stores your energy to use later. Normal human adults are estimated to consume around 1800 to 2000 Calories each day. They shouldn't eat less than 1500 Calories to prevent malnutrition.

There are three essential elements called macronutrients which your body requires in huge amounts. The body converts the macronutrients into fuel. These are fats, carbohydrates and proteins.

Carbohydrates, along with fats, are the body's primary energy source. Carbohydrates are generally called sugars, starches and fibers. Carbohydrates don't have to be sweet. Most everything is made of carbohydrates, like animals and plants. They usually provide around 4 Calories per grams.

Fats are similar to carbohydrates, but are better known as oils. They are not usually dissolved in water, unlike other carbohydrates. When people consume excessively, the body stores fat, which causes the person to gain weight. But, human beings can live without carbohydrates, which causes their bodies to burn calories instead of gaining energy.

It is referred to as ketogenic diet and although it might be beneficial, more studies are needed to determine whether consuming less carbohydrates can result in negative consequences. Fats provide around 9 calories per grams.

In the end, proteins are utilized by your body for building muscles along with other types of cells. They can be found in meats as well as in some plant-based products, like soya and nuts. In general, your body doesn't use the energy sources when there's anything else left. They provide around 4 calories per gram.

If you work out, then not just does your body become warmer because you use up your stored energy, but you also sweat. It's not just made of water. It also contains various mineral (or electrolytes) which your body requires. If you exercise it is important to ensure to replenish minerals and fluids to prevent dehydration or developing a health problem.

Drinks for sports contain essential nutrients to replenish your body, however they also contain a lot of sugar. An alternative is a mix of fruit juice and water.

The muscles of the skeletal system

The bones of our bodies support our entire body, which is the reason bones can be found from our head all the way to our toes. They shape our bodies. In freerunning and parkour the body's primary components required to perform the correct movements are the muscles of the skeleton. Muscles connect to bones via the tendons.

Muscles are comprised of tiny strings, referred to as muscle fibers. The components of the fibers move over one another and cause muscles to relax and contract. In order to help support movement, multiple muscles contract, and the other muscles work in tandem. This allows for fluid movement.

Because multiple muscles within one muscle group play a role for many body movements, one should be constantly training the muscles to be able to perform the execution. It should also be observed that coordination that occurs within the muscles themselves. Muscles decide which units they will use to ensure that they don't over-work the muscles.

There are two major types of the skeletal muscles. The first is the red or slow muscle. It is distinguished by a particular slow-twitch fiber, which is known as the Type 1. The slow-twitch fiber of the muscle allows muscles in the red to ward off exhaustion, and is crucial for supporting functions like standing.

The second kind of skeletal muscles is the white or fast muscle. White muscle is comprised of what is known as the Type 2-muscle fiber, which is focused on short bursts of movements such as running, jumping or landing. Due to this, white muscles get tired faster in comparison to muscles with red.

Everybody has muscle groups which possess two kinds of fibers. The difference between a person is the proportion of white and red muscle fibers. One thing is that this is controlled by genetics.

When your family members have more identified Type one muscle fibers due to of their endurance needs during work or other activities then you're likely to inherit the power of Type 1 . Muscle fibers. If, however, you did not start out with more Type 1 muscle fibers, you may develop the other kind of muscle fiber through regular training. This is that athletes in various sports have different proportions of muscles fibers.

As a potential freerunner or traceur you should ensure that you build the muscle fibers of Type 2. This will help your body to withstand tensions and shocks during intensive freerunning or parkour movements. It's a excellent start if have the right muscle structure for freerunning or parkour.

If this is not the scenario (and generally it isn't) It will give you an idea of that you can't think of performing certain movements when you are just in the beginning. It is essential to keep training your body and build the type 2 muscles prior to when you can move on to more challenging and advanced exercises.

Chapter 5: Understanding the Concepts of Training

It is the final chapter on the theories and the concepts that underlie parkour and freerunning. As a final point to be discussed prior to introducing the freerunning and parkour movements first, you need to understand the concept of exercising. This will assist you in how you can plan your workouts and the requirements to meet in order to be an effective freerunner or traceur.

Physical adaptation

The most fascinating aspects of our body's structure is the fact that it is capable to adapt and better respond to specific external stimuli. We've seen this at the classroom through the concept of evolution, where humans have evolved to improve its survival abilities.

Presently physical change is not yet being observed. Bodybuilders' muscles grow bigger to enable them to lift greater weights. The people who constantly wash their hands or any other work that is heavy will develop calluses to ensure that these tasks won't cause too much discomfort.

In our instance as freerunners or traceurs continuous training can allow our body to more effectively respond to the stimuli is exposed. Exposure to a stimulus that is too intense for our bodies can cause strains or other injuries. It is essential to take into consideration the strength of your body when you do freerunning or parkour. By lifting weights , or doing other exercises that improve our strength as well, our muscles, bones ligaments, joints and tendons improve their ability to cope those physical challenges of parksour or freerunning.

The science behind training

Since the recognition and understanding of science was developed as science, a variety of groups and individuals have been involved in giving objective standards to determine how to proceed when training. There are many factors involved when it comes to training. Every type of exercise is different based on your fitness objectives.

There are four major motor abilities that are acquired through various forms of exercise. These include endurance, strength as well as speed and flexibility. Based on the goals you wish to achieve or are looking to improve the training regimen will differ greatly. I'll go over with you the four most important motor skills and how you can enhance these.

Enhancing endurance

Endurance is the ability in performing for a prolonged duration of time. Although it may not be the most crucial skills in freerunning or parkour but it will aid in staying longer working on other skills. The endurance training method will teach your body to release energy over a lengthy period of time.

Running is the best method to improve endurance as it demands your body to continuously release energy. Beginners who haven't yet learned any other skills of motor are required to run. Professionals require more endurance training and so would prefer longer runs.

For beginners, it is recommended to do intense endurance runs at least 3 times per week. They are asked to run for between 30 and 60 minutes using a device that measures their heart beat. A treadmill can assist novices achieve this. The runner has to keep a heart rate between 140-160 beats per min (bpm) but this is the norm for 20-30 year olds, and can differ for different age groups.

Strengthening the body

Strength refers specifically to muscle strength which is the amount of muscle strength our muscles can exert. Therefore, it's important when it comes to parkour, as stronger muscles is also associated with better-conditioned joints. This helps us optimize our training and prevent injuries.

There are three kinds of strengths can be used in freerunning and parkour.

The first one, the maximal strength refers to the most strength that an individual can apply. The approach to training for this is to simply increase muscle. Beginning athletes can develop maximum strength by lifting 40-60 percent intensity, with between 8 and 12 reps for each set, which is an average of 4 to six sets. Lifting should be slow, and the time between sets must be between 2 and 4 minutes.

The other, speed strength refers to the ability to move your body at high speed. Because this requires rapid bursts of massive energy, it is not suitable for those who are just beginning. When you are skilled in maximum strength, the ideal speed workout routine will be performing exercises at 80-90 percent intensity, with three to six reps per set, which is for 6-8 sets. Lifting should be swift and the time between sets should be 3 to 5 minutes.

The third strength, called reactive refers to the capacity to swiftly adapt or convert energy. This will help freerunners and traceurs improve their jumps. For beginners, training should be 100% intense or more and with 6 to 10 reps each set, for an average of 2 to three sets. Lifting should be quick or explosive, and the time between sets must be 3 to five minutes. Make sure you don't injury yourself while working on the strength of your reaction. Always begin with maximal strength before working on this.

Improved speed

Speed is the capacity to give the fastest possible reaction to a movement in a particular scenario. It's all about the speed of fast-twitch muscle fibers. Training will then be concerned with making slow-twitch muscles fibers faster-twitch muscles fibers.

In contrast to the strength training I can't give you the intensity required to build the speed skills. Instead, the proper training environment must allow you for running at the maximum possible speed. This means that the individual who is training be completely dedicated and driven.

For each rep, the run is supposed to last for a long time so that at the end the participant will not be exhausted to the point of exhaustion. This means that performance won't be impaired. The remainder should be sufficient for a full recovery from previous workout, which could be 3-10 minutes or longer, depending on the individual.

Enhancing flexibility

Flexibility is the ability to perform a wide range of activities. Due to the requirements of freerunning and parkour it is among the most crucial abilities to develop. The goal of training is to increase the flexibility of muscles as well as the body as a whole to allow for greater movements.

For improving flexibility, stretching an most appropriate exercise. For those who are new to stretching, it is important to begin by warming up before stretching. This will prevent injuries. Then, stretch your legs until you feel discomfort. This is the maximum amount of your stretching and must not go beyond this. It is best to do these exercises in the afternoon or in the evening. In addition, contrary to what is commonly believed stretching actually increases muscle soreness. Consider this when performing any flexibility exercises.

Chapter 6: Running and Balancing

Before you are able to engage with roofs, walls and other types of surfaces it is essential to initially gain momentum when you come to them. This chapter focuses on keeping your balance and moving in the right way to be able to perform the movements in subsequent chapters.

Maintaining your balance

Balance is the most important and vital quality of parkour and freerunning. This is particularly apparent when athletes are on the top of bridges or structures. An incorrect estimate of balance could cause many issues.

There are two major types of balance. The static balance refers to the capacity to remain still. The second one, dynamic balance refers to the capacity to maintain the correct height during the course of movement.

In the first place, it's impossible for any human being to stand still for long periods of time. Contrary to rocks that are laid on top of each the other, human beings are amidst multiple complex machinery operating within their bodies, which hinder balance from being simple. For static balance, imagine a person standing on a tightrope. While trying to hold his place along the rope, they have to move his arms in order to stay in equilibrium. If he remained in a static position, it would be impossible to walk.

There are many ways of practicing static balance

1. One-legged stand. It is necessary to sit on one leg in front of a thin surface , such as the plank.

2. Laying down. Like the one-legged stand the procedure is simple. It requires you to lay down in a stomach position or on a surface that is narrow. This is crucial to ensure your balance when moving.

3. Handstands. All freerunners and traceurs should be able to hold a hand. For beginners, it is recommended to practice against the wall, and then gradually shifting towards it. The ability to perform handstands using one hand is essential to be safe.

4. The knees are bent and you sit in a squat position. This is a position that will require you to begin with a standing posture and slowly descend to the squat position while keeping your knees in a forward position. This will allow your knees to be able to carry heavier than they normally do.

To develop dynamic balance The above methods can be used while moving. The ability to balance dynamically is continuously honed through other freerunning or parkour exercise.

Take flight

It is not common for people to begin their performances by walking across a surface. Freerunning or parkour running is not just about speed, but it also requires the athlete to consider methods of removing obstacles in his way.

Training for running doesn't need the athlete to run over a vast area (unless you are doing endurance training). Parkour and freerunning generally calls for an initial sprint, then transition into a shorter run prior to getting to be able to communicate with the surface.

The issue with doing short distances of training is that it doesn't encourage good cardiovascular development. Although training for short distances will help you build the ability to balance, speed and flexibility in preparation for the actual thing, it completely ignores the need to utilize different body parts in real situations to perform freerunning or parkour moves.

Training for short distances does not permit your body to disperse energy in long periods (as in real life) because you're only focused on finishing a short course. This is that endurance training via running is essential. It can significantly increase the endurance of your workout through a delay in fatigue. It will also enable you to recover more quickly between training sessions or repetitions.

Chapter 7: Jumping and Landing

This chapter will focus on landing and jumping that, along with running and balance, constitute the fundamental movements in freerunning and parkour. Jumping is the action that is required in order for any kind of distance that is impossible to traverse with a single run or walk. It is also a way of covering gaps and heights. Landing is the process to recover from an leap and then returning to the ground or the surface. Unintentional landings can hurt the person who is performing.

There are three main kinds of jumps that are common in freerunning and parkour. They are taking-off jumps with tic-tac precise jumps, precision jumps, and drops. I will discuss each of them in depth. I will also offer specific landing ideas for each type of jump needs an exact landing method.

Tic-tac take-offs

Tic-tac-stepping movements are any type of movement that requires you to press against the wall. Take-offs with tic-tac are therefore requiring you to put the soles of your feet against the wall. The purpose of performing tic-tac take-offs is that you are raised.

These are the steps to follow to play the tic-tac

1. Watching the angles. Before you start running towards the wall, note the wall's side. In the case of a wall on your left, then you'll have to use your left leg to get to the wall. It is the opposite for walls on your right. After you've taken note of the wall then you could begin to run toward the wall.

2. Preparing. Your body should be tilted at around 45 degrees from the wall while you run. If you reach the wall, walk away with your foot away of the wall. You can then take the other foot and set it as far up the wall as is possible.

3. Pushing. At the center of your stride, your foot that is closest to your wall will touch it on the top of your foot. When the height of your foot is in your hips, apply pressure to forcefully push the sole of your foot to the wall. This will enable you to raise your foot further.

4. Maximizing. When you are in the air, bend your knees , and keep the legs in as tight as is possible. This will reduce the force of air and allow you to leap higher. Your torso must be strong and straight in a similar location in relation to the wall.

5. Landing. The landing you make will be contingent on the specifics of your tic-tac start. If you traveled a long distance, like through jumping over obstacles then you will have to align your two feet in order to utilize them both when your return back to earth. Smaller jumps could allow only one-foot landings , so you can transition to a different method, however for a beginner, it is best to be familiar with two-foot landings regardless of distance that you fly.

Precision jumps

In contrast to tic-tac jumps that concentrate on covering a huge height gap Precision jumps, instead, concentrate on landings that are calculated. This is essential for unstable surfaces like roofs with brittle areas as well as in risky platforms like narrow ledges.

There are three different ways to execute an accurate jump. The first method is the one-footed , precision jump. It's the most basic and least difficult to master. The majority of people use precision jumps with one foot to fill in small gaps. This technique isn't so well if the landing area is located at an elevation higher.

These are the steps to make one-footed precision jumps

1. Positioning. Place yourself on the ledge you'll leap off of. The ledge should be close to the area you wish to fall on.

2. Preparation. Take one leg and then swing your arms forward to back.

3. Take-off. As you move your hands in the direction of a forward motion, make use of this momentum and push your foot towards the ledge. This allows you to jump into the air. When you're in the air, extend your arms inwards. This will help you remain in balance during landing.

4. Landing. To ensure your stability, you'll need to make use of both feet when landing. Be sure your feet are equal distance from the surface your landing. As soon as your body comes into touch with the floor let your body be close to the surface. If you don't allow this, the force of gravity could push your

body forward and result in a trip or to fall.

The primary purpose behind one-footed precision leaps is to cover a small area. Naturally, using one foot to jumps would not permit your body push in a forward direction for too long. This offers some safety against miscalculations regarding distance. If your objective is to cover more space, a precision two-footed jump is better. It's quite like the one-footed precision jump and the distinction is only visible prior to take-off.

To accelerate further after a precision jump that is one-footed it is not enough to move your arms back and forward to generate momentum, but you must bend your knees in order to create springs. As your arms propel the body upwards, then you could make use of this momentum to force down on your heels by bending your knees in order to propel yourself in the sky.

Other aspects of the leap are like the precision jump with one foot. It uses two levels of feet for landing the ball, and the feet are first to reach the surface.

The most precise jump is the one that covers the largest amount of space. It's referred to as the running jump and is basically an unfooted jump created by running toward the edge. One foot is all that is required to start the jump, and everything is the same as the one-footed precision jump that is separated of the run. Better landings can be made by landing on a surface located at a lower altitude; it will permit you to move your body during the air in mid-air.

Drops

The final form of jumping technique is different from the tic-tac take-off and the precise jump. Instead of pushing the body upwards, drops are simply leaping down.

This kind of jump is the most simple type of jump you can perform after the one-footed leap. The most important considerations in drop jumps are the hight of the initial leap as well as the safety and accuracy of landing.

In the initial leap the leaps that are too high permit gravity to exert more force on you, which makes the fall more difficult and difficult to control. Be aware that, at high enough force, even two-foot landings will not be able to handle the fall. To ensure a safe landing one must keep his head up while keeping his eyes on his landing location.

The head should be raised to assist in stabilizing his motion in during the air, and it will not change his location. The landing distance is typically two feet for shorter drops. However, for longer drops, two feet should be performed first, then a roll following landing. This allows the momentum you've left within your body to spread across your legs.

Chapter 8: The Vaults

There's a specific kind of jump that because of its importance isn't treated as an actual jump, but instead as a distinct move by itself. Vaulting permits you to leap over obstacles that hinder your feet from your hips, and even up to your chest. I will go over two essential vaulting strategies in this section, specifically the step vault as well as the speed vault.

If you're looking for an easy move to use to push yourself over fences and similar obstacles The step vault is the technique that you should consider. Step vaults are distinguished by slow movement towards the obstacle, and then employing the obstacles as a support to move your body over it. Due to the motions it is only effective to obstacles which are higher than your hip. Here steps for performing a step vault

1. Approach. The obstacle is approached directly however depending on the obstacles you can also take a diagonal approach.

2. Preparation. Put either one or both hands upon the obstruction for assistance. When you are approaching the obstacle, ensure that you have one leg firmly grounded to the ground. This will be used to start your body.

3. Take-off. By using the ball of your foot that is grounded, propel yourself up. With your hand still resting on the obstacle to provide support then raise your leg so that you can be able to take a step backwards onto the obstacle. The leg that you are using to launch must not be in contact with the obstruction.

4. Landing. The leg you use to launch is the one that first that hits the ground. Because the other leg needs to be extended, you should position the leg so that it is directly in front of the launch leg. This will enable you to quickly transition to running.

It is possible to observe while watching professional shows they show that the step vaults don't feature a distinctive slow approach. If you've got enough practice, you'll achieve the same feat. Rapid approaches are the hallmark of transitions that occur from an exercise or landing.

If you are able to perform quick steps to the step vault the speed vault will be a breeze. It is performed as the course when you are faced by a small obstacle. The obstacle can still cause the running. It is similar to completing a hurdle. Here are the steps needed to do the speed vault

1. Preparation. Begin by running towards the obstacle. At the end of your running the right leg should be in good condition since this will serve to taking off.

2. Take-off. Then, push the right foot's heel against the floor. As you are in the air, bend your left leg , then raise your right leg. You can additionally kick your left leg to lengthen it. Place your right hand against the obstruction to provide support. Your body should be in line with the obstruction.

3. Adjustment. After your body has moved over the obstacle, but is suspended in mid-air, extend your right leg, then pull it towards the ground.

4. Landing. Your right leg should touch on the ground the first. You should bend your body forward when you touch the

ground. This will allow you to transition back into running.

Chapter 9: Climbing

The next move you can be covered is climbing. There are a few heights that can be covered with a tic-tac take-off because walls may not be in place. In the same way, you might not be able precise jumps on certain gaps that are too big or the landing zone is not stable.

For beginners climber, it is best to practice on surfaces that are near the ground. The best guideline is If you are unable to jump down, you should not climb up. Injury is very easily incurred when climbing, so be extra cautious.

This chapter I will introduce the most basic climbing techniques including the wall run as well as the arms jump.

Wall runs are an exercise that is used to swiftly climb over walls. This is due to the speed of your approach. You can use the speed of your running to allow your body to climb up the wall. You need to have sufficient muscle strength to to lift yourself up using just one arm. These are the steps needed to complete the wall run:

1. Approach. Take a stride towards the wall and be cautious not to be too close. You should be a distance from the wall prior to taking off.

2. Take-off. Place you foot's ball to the ground in order to leap up. Place your free leg on the wall. When your body is close to your wall hold it in a straight position and make use of your free leg to push against the wall and propel you up.

3. Climbing. Utilize the force that the leg pulls to climb to the highest point of the wall with one hand. Follow it with the other hand. If you are a beginner it is recommended to practice getting to the top using both hands since this will help you gain the stability you need. When your hands are resting on the wall, you should push your feet towards the wall. Once your chest is aligned with the wall's highest point Place your palms flat over the high point of the wall. Lift your body up.

4. Landing. One foot should be placed to one side. Once you are stable, straighten your body and pull the other foot up. The task is complete when you're standing straight against the

wall. You can do a drop for a move to the other side.

A wall-run is a basic and should be able to cover a variety of obstacles. But, there is situations that the distance is large or too far so that you can't make use of your feet as a support. In such a case you'll need to perform an arm leap. Here are the steps for performing an arm leap:

1. Take-off. To ensure stability, do not touch the platform unless essential. Take a leap from your position with either one or both legs. As you move your arms, swing them upwards towards the target. Once you're near move your legs up too.

2. Climbing. Your hands should be on the platform simultaneously with your feet are touching the side or the front of the platform (if there is one). Now you are hanging from the platform. Utilize your muscles and pull yourself up. For those who are new to the sport, practice in a place that you are able to fall when you can't get yourself up.

3. Landing. The landing is complete when you stand upright at the top of the step.

The wall run and arm jump, will provide the most basic challenges you will face in your first few years. Be sure to stay safe and practice more in this section prior to you proceed to the next chapter.

Chapter 10: The Swinging and Hanging

In the final section of the book I will teach you about swinging and hanging. These are two techniques you could be required depending on the circumstance. Due to the strength required for hanging and swinging I would suggest that you practice the techniques once you've learned the remainder of the book.

I'll focus on the lache. It in French is a way of letting go and let yourself go. In parkour, however lache is a term used to describe any method or movement that begins with hanging from your hands. The first time for a lot of people to experiment with lache was when they were they were playing on monkey bars on the playground, when they were young.

The idea of swinging and hanging best captured by monkeys that can effortlessly swing from branch to branch. Freerunners and Traceurs want to replicate this very attractive skill, even though we will never be able to fully imitate monkeys since our bodies are constructed differently.

Hanging and swinging are two of the most difficult exercises described within this publication. To execute the movements correctly it is essential that the individual has strong muscles in his arms, as well as physically strong shoulders and the torso. Additionally, the person must be able to balance well and have the flexibility to effectively swing and also be able to grip with a firm grip.

The first thing you should do in order to get yourself ready for in swinging and hanging is to improve your grip. When you decide to improve your swinging and hanging skills you're always working on your grip on the hand. If you have a weak grip, it can be dangerous as you may be thrown off balance and fall abruptly. Also being unsure of when to let go of your grip will result in the same disastrous consequences.

It is recommended to test these techniques in a gym where foams and bars are easily available. Security is the primary concern of any novice. If you don't have these facilities an erect railing or the strength of a tree branch may suffice.

Here are some tips to help you train swinging and hanging by improving hand grip:

1. Tighten your grip. For a beginner, you should repeatedly move your hands over the high branches of trees bars, edges, edges, or railings. This allows your hands to get used to the feel of the surface and prevent any accidents in the future in which you lose your grip because the surface is too rough.

2. Try swinging at a low level. The first time you try to learn swinging should be done at the smallest (but nonetheless elevated) edges, such as railings or branches. Repeat this process until you are confident with the idea. Be sure to be aware of your movements. You could push yourself forward too much. The force will propel you forward and create damage if the grip you hold isn't strong enough.

3. You can switch the direction. It is possible to work on to release your grip. It is only possible to do this in the moment that you are at the top position before you drop back down. This is due

to the fact that this is the point at which your speed is almost zero. In these instances you should try letting loose your grip, and then hold it back as you come back to the point of your fall.

4. Let go and come back. In real-life situations, you do have allow yourself to relax. When swinging, practice to make sure you catch your foot without falling or tripping. Through this exercise you will be able to determine when in your swing you can easily let go of your grip. This will help you improve your balance and enable you to develop your landing technique.

5. Target your landings. It's an important skill to know how to land by swinging. But the most crucial skill is to be able to land exactly that you would like to place your feet. To master this, you first mark the area you'd like to place your feet. It is more beneficial to envision your space as the actual situation, as some areas can be very risky to take a landing on. Practice by swinging your body to hit the spot you want to land on.

Each time you come across the edge of danger, take a look at your actions to determine what you can do to improve your. The majority of the time it will depend on the time you let go of your grip, as well as what the body's form was at the time you were hovering in midair.

Once you're comfortable with this technique Create a sturdy surface like a rigid crate , or horizontally stacked tops of boxes. This can be used to simulate real situations where the landing zone is made of a different substance that you'd imagine it to be.

6. Hang longer. One last thing you must do is practice holding onto the railing or the branch longer. This will improve the strength of your arms and endurance. This can be done as a complete workout in gyms through pulling-ups.

To build endurance To build endurance, you might begin by sitting still and then leaping to hang from the tree or a branch of a tree. Watch the moment you release. Perform two to three repetitions of this and try to maintain your initial pace. Do two to three minute breaks between reps. If you can comfortably complete the rep during your reps, add your time.

Another option is to hang from the run. This helps you prepare for situations in which you may require additional momentum to get to the bar. It will also teach you to control the force that propels you up the moment you are able to hold either the tree or bar. Similar to static training repetition, keep doing this until you are confident.

Once you've reached the level of mastery you desire then you can change it up by running up to an extended hang, then swinging until you land on a predetermined location. This can be a great way to train for urban areas. You could even allow your imagination to run wild and experiment with different environments.

Chapter 11: Define Free Running

Before proceeding, it's crucial to understand the meaning behind Free Running or Parkour is about. The definition of the term itself says, Free Running is being allowed to run in a free manner or without limitations. A different term used to describe Free Running, as provided by various websites, is that it is the ability for individuals to express themselves or herself through the freedom of movement.

A more in-depth definition about Free Running is defined as it is a type of martial art discipline that was first introduced in 2003, and was invented by Sebastien Foucan, a Frenchman from France. Free Running is synonymous to Parkour The main distinction between the two is the fact that Free Running has more acrobatic-like moves that are executed.

However, Parkour is a kind of training that utilizes exercises that are usually used in military training. The military personnel learn how to move from point A to point B efficiently and in the fastest

way possible using their body and their physical capabilities to get
there. Similar to Free Running, Parkour also was created within France and was created through Raymond as well as David Belle.

Free Running and Parkour both employ the fundamental movements that most people do, like running and swinging and climbing, jumping as well as rolling and vaulting. The movements mentioned above can be utilized in different combinations based on the environment accessible for the free Runner. So technically-speaking, Free Running and Parkour are one and the same.

Chapter 12: The Story of Free Running

While modern Free Running as well as Parkour could be attributed the work of Sebastien Foucan, the seed concept that led to the invention of Free Running and Parkour must be credited with Georges Hebert, a Frenchman who was an Naval officer in World War I. While he was within Africa, Hebert observed a specific tribe that had an athletic talent that was naturally present as no formal training was offered to their members at the time. Hebert observed the members of the tribe practice certain abilities that appeared to be quite advanced for their age, like easily climbing trees and leaping between rocks.

His insights led him to development of a distinct type of obstacle course which could be used to teach soldiers, dubbed"parcours du combattant" "parcours of the combattant". This type of military training presents a variety of challenges that soldiers must overcome using their bodies and physical capabilities.

"Parcours du combattant" consisted of ten core activities soldiers could use during training in self-defense, swimming lifting, balancing, throwing at, climbing, quadrupedal motion including jumping, running and walking. This method of training, devised by Hebert was the foundation for all training and education for military personnel during the war in France throughout World War I and II.

Alongside Hebert In addition, another name that has been connected to the development and growth of Parkour includes Raymond Belle and his son, David Belle. Raymond Belle, who was taken by his parents to an orphanage at the age of seven, trained for a long time to get stronger and to survive. Raymond was able to train secretly using the course used to train military personnel. However, once he was used to the challenges and hurdles created by the course, Raymond innovated by creating his own obstacle courses which could be utilized to test his physical capabilities and limits. Through this it was never tiring of preparing himself as every obstacle was a unique type of challenge which he had to overcome.

Raymond Belle's passion for Parkour carried over onto his younger son

David. The older Belle seemed to be influencing the young Belle by introducing her to Parkour however, in a different way as unlike his father the younger Belle was not interested in becoming a soldier. Fortunately, as David got older, he got curious about what his father did during his younger years and how the senior Belle was able to do such physically-challenging feats. The curiosity that he had generated made David to come up with his idea that he could develop new type of ability that could be applied in all aspects of life and not only in military training. So, the idea of modern-day Parkour was born. But , in contrast to his father's methods, David incorporated athletics and gymnastics into the strategies were developed by him.

David Belle, along with his companions, also enjoyed the idea of running, jumping and climbing walls. They formed a group dubbed the Yamakasi. The Yamakasi group practiced for many years before 1997 when Parkour began to gain traction and resulted in the group's being asked to a variety of occasions to take part in. Frenchman, Sebastien Foucan, the creator of Free Running was part in the group Yamakasi.

After the group had was able to decide to part ways, methods, continued development for Parkour would be inevitable. Sebastien Foucan saw the chance to further develop Parkour as a more individual sport that one could engage in to express self, not an activity that groups of people perform frequently. The vision of Foucan can be compared to the reasons that made legendary martial artist Bruce Lee create Jeet June Do. Foucan started developing his own style of training which was influenced by Belle and transformed it into a new type of sport. Then, in 2003, the sport that is Free Running began.

As we mentioned previously, Free Running and Parkour are the same thing. The only distinction between them is the concept that the creators had in their minds at the time when they created the process. The first was created through David Belle as his tribute to his father's legacy. Sebastien Foucan invented the second to express himself.

Chapter 13: The Philosophy of Free Running

Free Running is not only about testing physical limits without limiting one's movements. Free Running has a more important goal beyond it's primary purpose. Belle and Foucan developed Parkour and Free Running because they also wanted to establish an idea that can be utilized in everyday life by those who share the same philosophy like them.

The underlying philosophy behind Free Running is the belief that man ought to be at ease with ease and without limitations in his movement. This is the philosophy Foucan wrote in his book on Free Running. In the work, Foucan mentioned a number of philosophical ideas that could be applied to understand the art in Free Running. Fundamentals like the ability to overcome any obstacle , and understanding competition as a limit and an illusion are a few aspects Foucan discusses in his book named, Free Running. Implementing these concepts will not only help you become an effective participant in Parkour but it will help you become a stronger, more confident and confident person.

However, aside from the philosophical ideas of Foucan the other principle that people who participate in who practice Parkour as well as Free Running follow is an concept proposed by Daniel Llabaca who said that people should be encouraged to think positive simply because Llabaca stated that those who think that they will likely fall are more likely to fall than people who believe that they will be successful. Being positive in your thinking decreases the likelihood of falling. Simply put, if think that you'll fall, it is likely that you'll fall, however, if you believe that you won't fall, the odds of falling are much lower.

Since its inception There have been numerous ideas and concepts established by Parkour followers. One of these principles is the concept that is "human regeneration". Human reclamation can be defined as the process to regain the humanity of a person. It implies that man must be able to travel from one location to another using the basics of what were taught to us in the beginning of the age of infancy.

The idea was born out of the tendency of people to be dependent on modern-day means of transportation to take them to places they'd like to go. In addition, the advent of skateboards and bicycles led to many people dependent on them instead of making use of their feet and hands to travel. The concept that "human reclamation" suggests that you don't require skateboards or bicycles to get your to the places you would like to travel. All you really require to do is use your body. You can utilize your feet and hands to get you where even skateboards and bikes can not.

Furthermore, Parkour can provide a innovative and distinctive way for people to engage with the urban landscape. There is no stadium or arena that is required to engage in Parkour. Your entire surroundings are your field. You are able to do anything and anything you like in your environment. Through Free Running, the sky is the limit, both literally and metaphorically talking.

Chapter 14: Free-Run Movements

When it comes to Free Running There are any official lists of Parkour actions other than most basic moves that men are able to perform, like jumping, running and climbing, for example.

In order to be successful to be successful Free Running, you must be aware of your body's physical abilities and limitations. It is important to be aware of what you can and cannot accomplish. If you do this it will be simpler to adapt to what kind of movement you are able to perform securely.

Free Running does not require any particular physical capabilities in the event that you can do the basic moves that nearly everyone can perform. The trick is to combine the movements that transfer you body position to another.

The the early fans of Parkour have created various styles that are currently being practiced by current fans. Every style comes with its unique distinct set of moves, and that's what differentiates each style in comparison to the other styles.

To help you gain an idea of the nature of these essential Free Running movements, visualize how these examples are performed by Parkour athletes. You can also watch videos on the internet. These are:

The Run-Jumpp-Push combination

This kind of move is performed when you wish to get to the top of the wall easily.

The Vault

This kind of move is used when you need to overcome obstacles of high height like stairs, walls and fences.

The Roll

This type of motion is performed when you wish to reduce the force of a fall. This is because the rolling motion can help to absorb the impact point.

It's the Jump & Catch

This type of maneuver can be done when trying to get through an extremely narrow or small obstruction.

Understanding these fundamental Free Running movements is the first step you need to master if you wish to master Free Running properly and safely. You can easily discover great videos for these movements by searching for the appropriate keywords on Youtube.com!

Chapter 15: The Risks of Free Running

When you engage in any sport that you choose to play there are going to be some risk involved. For security and safety reasons it is essential to be aware of the dangers you might face prior to engaging in any kind of physical activity in nature.

The athletes who participate in Free Running can encounter a number of hazards, however those who participate in Free Running are usually subjected to two primary kinds of risk that include injuries and trespassing. The first kind of risk is more about logistical issues that you may confront, while the other kind of risk is the more personal issue because it has an immediate impact on the individual who is practicing the sport. It is important to note that injuries could be fatal and end careers too.

Trespassing can be a crime under the law when you are in a location which you cannot gain access to the area, unless you are granted the express permission of. The people who practice Parkour are usually found guilty of trespassing as they are typically observed Free-Roving in public areas without getting permits from the relevant authorities.

It is generally accepted that Parkour shouldn't be performed in public areas such as playgrounds or parks. There have been some attempts by some to build places that Parkour fans can practice their sport with safety and in a proper manner. But , those efforts have been delayed because the concept of creating a space specifically for Parkour is in contradiction to its basic principles of innovation, adaptability and the freedom.

The past has seen Parkour users have found in both urban and rural places like offices, gyms or even abandoned buildings. The majority of the time the public has expressed their concerns about possible violations individuals who engage in Free Running can commit.

Because Free Running is a means to express oneself, those who practice Free Running sometimes forget that being a self-expressionist is not without limitations in relation to the laws. Although it's the truth that you shouldn't permit yourself to be restricted to the places you can go to perform your sport However, making sure you're not in violation of the law must not be overlooked.

The best way to stop you from being a trespasser is easy - get an appropriate permit from authorities prior to leaping, climbing, or walking around the streets.

There are also locations that aren't suitable for the practice of Parkour due to safety or other factors. Cemeteries and airport terminals shouldn't be used as places that allow Free Running because it is not appropriate and there are significant security concerns associated with it. Like in every similar sport, the safety is the first priority, particularly in the case of not being professionally paid to play.

In addition to trespassing, another type of risk that participants of Parkour typically have to face is being injured. Some who oppose this form of Parkour assert that those who participate In Free Running pose a high chance of inflicting injury to themselves. The majority of injuries happen when the movement isn't properly executed or the setting isn't sturdy or secure.

As they say, accidents are a part of growing older. If you don't suffer injuries then you won't be able to learn from your mistakes and you'll be unable to adjust your actions to help you to avoid repeating the same mistake again. Accidents are inevitable, particularly due to the physical demands of Parkour. Speeds that are extremely high as well as jumping from one rooftop to the next and climbing walls can be dangerous at any time in the event that you don't properly prepare and assess.

Since it is not possible to stop injuries from occurring The best thing you can do is to be prepared mentally, physically, and emotionally to ensure that, if the moment comes when you do suffer an injury you're prepared to manage the injuries.

Chapter 16: Free Running Equipment

In general, there's no set of equipment or clothing needed to practice Parkour. However, practitioners typically wear clothes that they are comfortable in. Wear whatever you want in the event that you can be able to move comfortably and freely within it. Do not wear clothing that make you feel constrained particularly when you spread your legs.

Also, having a quality set of shoes for runners that are comfortable to wear and provide adequate traction can be beneficial. Presently various shoe manufacturers such as Nike have developed shoes specifically designed specifically for Parkour.

Certain companies have gone the extra mile and begun to explore the possibility of making different products that can be utilized to facilitate Free Running. In the last few months, some manufacturers of sports equipment have come up with a new kind of sports glove with an extremely thin surface. This is the kind of glove you use in order to safeguard your hands and offering the best grip on anything you are holding.

When it comes to Free Running, style is all that matters, while self-expression is the most important thing. You are able to go Free Running without any clothes on if you want to be a way to express your personality .... provided you're not violating any laws.

Chapter 17: The Development of Free Running

Since the idea of Parkour was first introduced by Hebert in World War I, Free Running has certainly increased in its popularity. In the past, Parkour was just limited to the military , however with the years, Parkour has gotten out of the world of military service and has become a part of the lives of the general public.

In the present, a rising amount of individuals are expressing interest in what's currently thought to be an extreme sport across many regions around the globe. The rise of Free Running can be attributed to the efforts of its founders to make people know about the existence of Free Running.

The year 2003 saw a film starring Parkour called Jump London, was aired on the public television. The documentary revealed the basics of what Parkour was all about as well as how it got started. Then, at the end of the documentary, Sebastien Foucan, together with his colleagues Parkour teammates, Johan Vigroux and Jerome

Ben Aoues showed off their abilities in Parkour. Jump London jump started Free Running's popularity in the current period.

In the wake of Jump London's popularity Other documentaries on Parkour were produced like Jump Britain in 2005. Also on September 16th in 2007, Foucan along with Vigroux were featured in an episode that included Parkour in an Australian version of 60 Minutes.

However, the rise of Free Running wasn't only because of the television. There's been many films which feature Parkour. In the film Taxi 2, which was presented in 1998. There was a scene that featured Parkour participants participating in a chase scene. In 2001 Luc Besson, a popular French director, produced the film Yamakasi which featured nearly all of the original core members of the organization. The year 2004 saw a follow-up to Yamakasi was released through the movie Les fils du vent.

Besson was so fascinated by Parkour that he made a second film on Free Running that starred Cyril Raffaelli and David Belle. The film's name is Banlieue

13, which means District 13 in English. Five years after, Besson again produced a sequel titled District 13: Ultimatum.

Free Running's popularity within films wasn't just restricted in feature-length films. The mainstream film industry of Hollywood produced films that featured Parkour like movies like The Bourne Ultimatum and James Bond's Casino Royale. Actor Aamir Khan was required to master Parkour during shooting Dhoom 3, which was released in 2013.

In video games too influences of Parkour cannot be ignored. There are games with game elements that incorporate moves that are associated with Free Running. The video game, Assassin's creed several of the major game characters such as Altair, Connor, and Edward employ Parkour throughout the story. Also, in a video game that features Tony Hawk, Tony's character employs several Free Running movements when he isn't on his skateboard.

Chapter 18: Future of Free Running

Free Running certainly has an exciting future. As the sport is slowly growing in acceptance across the world particularly on the Internet There will be the time that Parkour will be recognized in areas of the world which aren't aware of it.

The concept behind Parkour has seen a number of changes since the first time it was thought of. What began as a basic training tool used by military soldiers has transformed into a means to express yourself.

Free Running has certainly increased in popularity and will only continue to increase in the event that more people are interested in it. Don't be deceived by the ease with which Free Runners make the sport appear. On paper, it could appear simple to perform however to actually practice it requires effort, dedication, and training. Because of this, there will always be a large number of people watching the YouTube videos as opposed to those that actually play the sport. The "awe" aspect of this game will likely remain the same.

If there's one thing that is certain about what's to come from Free Running that some people tend to overlook that is that Parkour is a great choice as a method for weight loss. Free Running offers all the necessary elements for an effective workout routine, including aerobic exercise, muscle building and tone your body. Running continuously, climbing walls and moving between platforms is sure to make you sweat. The best part of it all is you are able to run at your own speed and at your own time. It's a great method of losing weight since you're utilizing your surroundings to aid in losing weight and increase your confidence.

Chapter 19: Define Parkour and Freerunning

You've heard of it and probably have seen the show on TV or on the internet. There's something very magnetic about running and parkour which may be the reason you decided to purchase this book. People who do their sport run straight lines, yet their movements remain fluid and angular.

It is no wonder that the sport of freerunning and parkour has attracted those in need of adrenaline and those who are enthralled by the excitement of witnessing the splendor of human athleticism.

But what exactly is the differences between parkour and free running? What is the difference between the other?

Parkour is concerned with the effective coverage of pathways. The person who is a parkourer, known as traceur (which literally means one who tracks the path) is able to reach a different point that is completely free of the expectations of culture and architecture. If there's a winding road that connects two points, you should not think that a traceur simply follow the route laid out by the road.

In this way the traceurs' abilities, they decide for himself which route to follow so that he is able to easily overcome any obstacle they may encounter along the way. The primary goal of the parkour world is speed as well as speed of execution There isn't a right or wrong way to go the ability to masterfully control one's body on the shortest distance between points is the ultimate goal that the traceur strives for. Everyone who traceurs wants to understand the most effective method of moving between points.

Freerunning is regarded as an adaptation of parkour. Instead of being focused on moving forward in order to cover a route the focus of freerunning is the flexibility and creativity of the body. Freerunners look for ways to be creative and personal connect with their surroundings by moving. Although the goals are different, the basic movement patterns and strategies that are used in parkour establish the foundations of freerunning.

Incredibly, however the growing acceptance of freerunning has led to the development of a variety of new moves in an hour. Because the focus is to show off Acrobatic elements from a variety of disciplines have inspired freerunners. In urban settings, freerunners have utilized gymnastics techniques and extreme martial arts. breakdance, and Capoeira that is an Brazilian combat art.

Since freerunning allows the runner to express themselves and be completely free exhibitions are always fresh to offer, as freerunners use a an array of different moves.

Both freerunning and parkour have seen an enormous increase in popularity due to the internet. The capacity of online streaming sites to show exhibitions in freerunning and parkour and tutorials has let the young people from across the globe to participate and learn about the sports. If there's a passion in freerunning or parkour there will be a local community that can always be found. The internet has enabled many people to join and even encourage individuals to form national teams that participate in official competitions.

However, both parkour and freerunning are an excellent fitness and leisure sport. You don't need to perform extreme stunts or compete in international contests to take pleasure in and appreciate the sport.

Chapter 20: American Ninja Warrior Competition

The American Ninja Warrior obstacle course competition is a tv show which has been broadcast on NBC since the year 2009. The series was launched as a spin-off from Sasuke literally translates to "Excellence" which has been held in Japan from 1997. Sasuke has become a global phenomenon as 100 participants include postal workers, fishermen doctors, teachers and carpenters who train throughout the year and put their jobs in a bind to compete for complete victory, or "kanzenseiha" in the mountains of Mount Midoriyama. In the course's 2,900 attempts, only three people have won Kanzenseiha (One person has won twice). Each time a person is named champion, the course is completely revised.

Since the beginning of the show seven spin-offs across different countries were developed that included the show on NBC called "American Ninja Warrior" (NBC owns G4 which is the channel that broadcasts Sasuke). In order to be eligible for the top prize of $500,000, contestants must complete four challenging stages, each more difficult than the one before. The event culminates in the final phase, Mount Midoriyama staged in Las Vegas, which consists of a strenuous rope climb. In the end, all participants in the American Ninja Warrior will then take part in Sasuke to face Japanese competitors.

The original American Ninja Warrior Competition was held in Japan's Mount Midoriyama after a series of qualifying events in Los Angeles; but since 2012, the location has changed into Las Vegas, Nevada, with a temporary Mount Midoriyama, as the producers believed that taking all participants to Japan every year was too demanding, both literally and metaphorically.

These are the Stages for the Contest

The tournament is made up of four stages that increase in difficulties. The obstacles are constructed on metal structures , with water beneath to absorb the impact in case a participant fall. To pass the stage and move on to the next one, the obstacles must be conquered without falling. This might sound more simple than it really is. Anyone who has seen the cult TV series will realize that not just pure power, but a lot of flexibility endurance, endurance and mental stamina are necessary to make it through the stage.

Stage 1. In this stage, competitors race against each other to achieve the fastest 30 times so that they can advance to stage 2. Although in Japan only 100 contestants are allowed to compete, American Ninja Warrior has no set a limit to the number of competitors who can participate on this course. Certain obstacles are different each season, but the most frequent obstacles in stage 1 include the "Jumping spider", "Half Pipe Attack" and "Warped Wall". A strong core is essential throughout the stages, but stage 1 demands you to be balanced and have flexibility.

Stage 2. The stage in which competitors do not just battle against one another however, they must also be able to compete against the race itself through more difficult obstacles than on the previous stage. The top 15 competitors will go on to the next stage. The main obstacles to be faced in this section include those of the "Double Salmon

Ladder", "Unstable Bridge", "Balance Tank", the "Metal Spin" and the "Wall Lift". Apart from the essential strength of the core, a lot of attention should be put on stability and leg strength.

Stage 3. This is where the majority of athletes fail, and go back to their homes to train intensely for the coming season. Stage three requires a huge upper body strength, and of course, core strength. Some of the most difficult obstacles include "Pipe The Jungle", "Ultimate Cliffhanger", "Doorknob Grasper", "Floating Boards" and "Little Dragons" "Spider Flip" and the absurd "Flying bar".

Before we get into the most effective preparation methods, let's first consider how to apply for American Ninja Warrior.

Chapter 21: The Application Process

The application process for every period of the American Ninja Warrior Competition happen two months prior to the start of the tryouts. They are held in:

* Pittsburgh, Pennsylvania

* Orlando, Florida

* Kansas City, Missouri

* Venice Beach, California

Go to http://www.adeignco.com/AmericanNinja Warrior/ to apply to compete on the show. On this website , you'll be able to find submission deadlines, regional qualifiers, and the final.

If you're located far from the venues listed above however, you can submit an application available on the website above. Then you'll be advised by the producers which location to audition, which is probably the one closest to you or where they think is suitable. Two phases in regional qualifiers that are "qualifiers" as well as "finals". Finalists from these regional championships play in Las Vegas, Nevada, to determine who will play at Mount Miyodori in Japan for Sasuke.

Requirements

* If you'd like to test something it, make sure you're

* Must be at the age of 21;

* A resident of the United States, and is legally resident in the country.

* No charge during the times and dates of auditions;

Make sure you are in top condition and you are able to take part in exhausting and demanding exercises, and

* Willing to submit a 2 to 3 minute video introducing yourself together with your clear digital photo and application details to http://www.anwcasting.com/, so you could qualify.

Complete the online application completely and without mistakes. Make sure that your friend reads it through before pressing"Submit. Your video submission is very crucial. Be sure to read the tips below carefully:

Create a motivational video. Make yourself known to the camera as well as the producers. You'll be on television! Naturally the producers are searching for outstanding personalities as well as great athletes. Discussing an inspiring life experience or having a fascinating hobby or interest, demonstrating your job as a commercial diver, salmon fisherman, or other interesting tale about your life will play an important factor in deciding if you're a good fit as a contestant. You'll be selected by the TV producers and this means that good personalities often be able to win over athletes who are good.

Be energetic. Be passionate about your training regimen or your town, your private life, your spouse or girlfriend and so on. Making sure you film every aspect of your life as well as your training, and displaying your pride in your hometown has been an important element in making a memorable video submission.

Make a quality video. Do not submit a video you shot with the new iPhone 6. I'm not trying to downplay the latest iPhone but having great lighting and a tripod for smooth and steady video recording, clear audio, and perhaps some innovative editing could make a difference.

After you've submitted your online application together with your high-quality inspiring video, let's concentrate on your workout routine and proper nutrition to help you get through the four phases.

Be aware that even though you aren't selected for the show, you'll be able to "walk through" during the day of regional qualifying. Plan to show up at least a week in advance and bring a companion and the tent. You'll need to ensure you reserve your place in the first ten persons waiting in line.

Chapter 22: the American Ninja Workout

Disclaimer 1: The workout plans and exercises are difficult and range between intermediate and advanced. This book isn't designed to help you go all the way from couch-to American Ninja champion and assumes that you're already in good physical shape. These exercises are designed to complement or replace your training routine to help increase endurance and build the proper muscles that can enable you to conquer the obstacles.

Disclaimer II: It is important to warm your body prior to engaging in. Begin by doing a 10 minute light run, cycle or run. Do a thorough stretch of your muscles and especially those which will be utilized (actively as well as passively) in your workout. You should allow at least 20 to 30 minutes to warm up , and be careful not to get injured. A sprain could cause you to miss several months, and may hinder your participation in the competition.

Disclaimer III The following work out routines assume that you have a an understanding of the basic terms used in exercise. Some workouts are dependent on climbing and employ terms such as "slopers Frenchies, crimps etc. If you're unfamiliar with a particular phrase, you should research it yourself and make sure you understand the workout before you attempt it.

I'm guessing that in reading this book, you're committed to doing the time and energy to improve your fitness. There is no shortcut to succeed in completing a stage or even achieving the title of champion. Before you go to the gym to begin working out, you must start by creating an overall training program. Instead of focusing on building general muscle mass, you should begin by focusing on specific areas like:

* Core strength overall

* Grip force

* Brachiate the monkey to can swing between branches

* Strengthening the upper body with explosive force

* Obstacles training

* Footwork

* Balance

If you've been following past seasons on American Ninja Warrior, you might have noticed two kinds of athletes perform very well: parkour and rock climbers.

The first thing you should do is to sign up with the rock climbing gym that has a the bouldering area or parkour gym. It is ideal to have the facility to exercise. Otherwise, sign up to an exercise gym.

You should exercise at least five, and preferably at least six times per week. Then, alternate one week with five working out days, and the next week with six working out days. It is essential to take your days off and to not become "over-trained" and result in injuries including stress fractures and tears in muscles. Injury is less likely to happen when you're not putting too much stress on your body, and avoidance of injuries is of the utmost importance in order to avoid setbacks in your training.

The ideal situation is to be able to access obstacles in your parkour facility or at home in your backyard. It is possible to purchase inexpensive blueprints of American Ninja Warrior obstacles online and then build the toughest ones, like those like the Salmon Ladder, Cliffhanger and Jumping Spider. It is a great way to practice the moves required for every obstacle. We'll go over each obstacle later.

Be healthy! This does not mean eating five hamburgers or eating a McDonald salad. It's true that having the correct diet is as crucial as having a strong physique. We'll discuss this in a future chapter.

You'll then see an example work out plan to ensure that you are prepared for any difficulty you'll encounter. Be sure to set small goals. By adding one more pull-up or a step higher, or climbing a grade higher. can help keep you focused throughout your training.

Be aware that you should be in good health. If you have doubts then you should first visit your physician to be approved for the intense workout program that is in place. I repeat the disclaimer above that I'm assuming you're reasonably healthy and have visited an exercise facility from inside before. If you find some exercises difficult or you aren't able to complete the suggested number of repetitions or sets, don't be concerned. Perform as many of them of them as possible. Through repetition of these exercises and remaining committed, you'll rapidly become stronger and fitter. Before every workout, warm up with a treadmill or a cycle as well as stretch the muscles minimum 15 minutes (shoulders fingers, forearms chest, back legs, abs, and legs).

It is important to note that for those who are brand novice to rock climbing and are not sure how to prepare, you must plan at least three months of training time, since you'll have to develop basic strength and technique prior to moving on to the next advanced to intermediate workouts. When you have signed for an account with a rock climbing club you should sign up for one or two climbing classes and begin working towards mastering the bouldering challenges. Bouldering can help you develop strong, dynamic core strength for the overhangs as well as grip strength on different kinds of holds.

The Schedule

Monday

AM: Run an early 5-8 mile run.

If you live in forests or other unpaved trails, I strongly suggest that you run cross-country and jump over tree stumps avoid snakes and rocks as well as avoiding branches, and then going downhill, trying not to slide. The exercise will boost your endurance, but will also significantly improve your feetwork.

Utilize a heart rate monitor to ensure that you are within 70 percent and the 80% mark of your training area (to to be determined following the below guidelines) to avoid you from depleting your body's glycogen reserves, making sure that you have enough strength to complete an intense exercise in the afternoon. To calculate the ideal heart rate for running you must first identify the different work-rate zones for your heart. Then, utilize these zones to help guide the pace you run at. The first step you have to do to do this is identify two crucial factors.

Your heart's maximum rate (MHR) is the most rapid rate your heart can beat every minute. To determine this rate you need to subtract one-half of the age you are from of 205. To test yourself on yourself, perform interval exercises, most preferably on a hill that is at least 300 or 200 yards or meters. Run up the hill, then run back down. Do this without stopping, repeat the sequence for five to six times and you'll likely reach an MHR that is at or near to your MHR. If there is no hill, you might want to increase the duration of your intervals by 400 meters.

The Resting Heart Rate (RHR) is the amount that you heart beats, when totally relaxed and free of extreme external stimuli such as the sound of loud music, caffeine or an illness that is on the horizon. In contrast to your MHR which can be fixed it is a measure of your overall fitness. It decreases slowly when you are physically fit. In general, the RHR of each person will vary significantly. Individuals who are not active might have a RHR in the vicinity of or above 100 beats per min. The majority of endurance athletes will be able to run at a pace below 60 to 50 beats per minute and at times, even under 40 beats per min. The lowest RHRs are those of elite runners, with some that fall under 30 beats per min. The reason for the slow heart rate of fit individuals is that the volume of stroke is so large that every heartbeat is able to pump around twice the amount of blood as those of an inactive adult. The heart rate is able to drop significantly but still providing the whole body with sufficient blood flowand oxygen. A heart that has a significant stroke volume indicates that it's a healthy heart that is resulting from an increased amount in aerobic endurance.

The best method of determining your RHR is to put to your monitor for heart rate early in the morning and before you get out of the bed. A simple lie-in for about two or three moments will provide you with an exact estimate of your heart rate.

You are now able to determine your training zones and create your personal chart that outlines the amount of strain you're placing onto your heart, at a certain rate. By using the following formula make a chart using increments of 5% all the way to 100%, which is your MHR.

((MHR-RHR) x Percent Level) + RHR

As an example, if that your MHR is 180, and you have a RHR of 85. your calculation for a percent level is:

((180-85) x 95%) + 85 = 175 beats per minute

Do this calculation for 90 percent and 85%, then 90%, 80%, and until you reach 5percent and then RHR. Take note of the results on the chart, which can help you with your training plan.

PM: Later in the afternoon go to the local rock climbing gym and then do the following workouts.

1. Begin by warming up with a simple rock climb, going upwards and down a few times.

2. Do 100 crunches, as well as 4 sets of Jack Knives

3. For the crunches lay on your back. Set your feet with shoulders wide apart. maintain your back straight on the ground . As you ascend exhale slowly, focusing on the abdominal muscles that are tight.

4. To do the Jack Knives For the Jack Knives, lay on your back and flat, stretch your arms outwards and raise your legs and arms up at the same time. Make sure you are touching your ankles with your arms extended and maintain a steady, well-controlled posture.

5. Go towards the hanging board (If you're able to afford $80, buy your hands on the Metolius Simulator 3D Training Board or the Metolius Rock Rings, which will give you a massive increase in grip strength as well as finger strength) Do the following:

* 5-10 Deadhangs for 5-10 seconds on

* Crimps

* Pinches

* Slopers

* Pockets

6. You're now warmed up for the 100 pull-ups workout.

* 8 Frenchies Each Frenchie comprising

* One complete pull-up Lock off for five seconds, then continue to go down

* With your feet not resting, or getting your feet on the ground, perform another pull-up until you are up, and then lock your arms in a 45-degree angle.

* With your feet not resting or getting your feet on the ground, perform another pull-up to the fullest extent up and secure your arms in 90 degrees.

* With your feet not resting, or getting your feet on the ground, perform another pull-up until you are up and secure your arms in a 120-degree angle.

* 8 times 6 uneven pull-ups. Four sets on each side.

* With one hand that is at five inches or more than the other hand Perform six pull-ups.

* Repeat this with the opposite hand, higher

* 20 pull-ups that are regular.

* Keep your hands locked for a few seconds, then slowly lower your body.

7. Then, you can finish by doing a campus workout. It is imperative to exercise extreme caution before beginning this exercise routine, because you may cause injury to your muscles. This is a challenging exercise

that should only be performed after you've gained solid finger strength.

* Ladder. Climb the board on campus as a ladder, using both hands on each rung moving both ways.

* Bumps. You can bump one hand up two rungs, then return to the ground, and then push the opposite hand up.

* Lock-Offs. Increase one hand until you are unable to go any higher before coming to a stop. Next, move the second hand up.

Double Clutches. This is where you push both hands on one rung at once moving up and down the board of the campus.

Training on campus, though difficult on your tendons will guarantee you gain insane finger strength , and you can take on the Cliffhanger hurdle without difficulty.

8. Hanging rock ball, the like similar to Cannonball Alley obstacle. If your gym is equipped with these tiny demons and you want to make use of these. These

are grapefruit-sized balls that hang on two straps.

* Grab both rocks and, while locking an arm extend the second one until it is fully extended Repeat this 10 times per arm.

* Lock one arm off by releasing it using the other. Switch hands, repeating 10 times.

* Finish with one Frenchie

9. If you're still not exhausted in the moment, you can finish off the day by having an exciting climbing session with your buddies.

Tuesday

This is an active day for climbing. Go to your rock climbing facility and begin to warm up on a bicycle or treadmill and move your muscles, focusing on your forearms, fingers and fingers. You can also perform some pull-ups.

I personally enjoy warming my fingers by climbing up a few walls using the "Autobelay" system. However, you could also attempt an easy traverse or simple problem with boulders. The key thing to remember is to select the climb that you are warming up on with a large hold.

You can increase the difficulty of your bouldering problems until you get to your maximum. Try tackling a few challenges to discover new moves as well as improve your hand-foot coordination and enjoy
yourself. Continue to pound until your hands and forearms are screaming.

Start climbing boulders and traversing walls until you are literally falling
off. Make sure you build your endurance at least one hour of climbing.

Perform 100 push-ups. You can alter them by using push-up handles, putting the feet upon a bench or TRX bands.

End your day by drinking the most Frenchies as you can .

Wednesday

AM: Do an early 5-8 mile run.

PM: Go into the fitness center, get warmed by stretching and warming up.

1. Begin by warming up with a simple climb up and down five times

2. Be prepared for 4x4s that consists in climbing 4 sets of boulders in succession. The sets are separated each time by a four minutes of rest. This exercise will help build your anaerobic endurance. This is crucial in the third stage of the American Ninja Competition. The routine will be repeated each week for a period of time up to your competition day.

The first thing to note is that this is a hard workout and will have you in a tense state. Make sure you push through your discomfort and give it your all.

Choose four boulders that are within you "onsight" maximum, that is, the grade you are able to typically climb in the first try but not be too difficult.

* Repeat the problem four times in succession, without stopping.

* Rest for four minutes, then continue with the next challenge by climbing the hill four times one row.

* Finish each of the four boulder challenges It should take about 25-30 minutes.

Your mind is focused on the future, and let go of the feeling of being "fit" as well as "in shape" you're seeking to exceed the level of fitness.

3. You should feel exhausted and nearly finished. We'll do a couple of leg exercises. It's the Bulgarian Split Squat and One Leg Deadlift, and the one-legged Squat

* To perform this exercise, the Bulgarian Split Squat, grab two dumbbells of 20 pounds as well as a knee-high stool which should be placed behind your back. Take one leg and then rest the other on the stool while you hold the dumbbells with your hands, and then squat down while making sure that your knee doesn't go over the shin or your back knee is almost touching the ground. Do three repetitions of between 8 and 12 reps each knee.

*The Single Leg Deadlift works stability and balance. Hold two 20-30lbs dumbbells with your hands. sit on one leg, while lowering the dumbbells onto the other side of your body. Bend the knee, pushing your forward with your hips while balancing the other leg. Make sure you keep the weight of your heels. Perform four sets on each leg.

*The Single Leg Squat involves standing on one leg , doing squats, and then you are balancing your other leg in front. Keep your weight on your heel and your shins in an straight line.

4. If you have gas left, you can end your training by bouldering your buddies and trying to solve certain difficult bouldering issues.

Thursday

It's your free day. Take a break from the tough days of training. Take in lots in food and drink plenty of fluids and take some sleep. Get up early to prepare for the next day.

Friday

This is a repetition of the Monday's workout. To spice things up instead of running you can opt to exercise Parkour or mountain biking or swim. It's crucial to change between your routines to ensure that you do not get tired mentally and keep your focus on the end target. Do the Hang-Board exercise 100 Pull-Up Workout Campus Board, and Rock Balls.

Saturday

1. Climb. Climb. Climb. Concentrate on the general climbing technique and tackle more difficult problems. Begin with a one-hour session, then go to the gym.

2. Do your best to strengthen your abs and core. Pick three of the exercises listed below and perform 4 sets of each Abs Wheel The Arms High Partially sit-up Leg Raise, Dip Combo, Plank, Side Plank medicine Ball Russian Twist and Legg Raises, Hanging Legg Raises. TRX Snaps, Jack Knives.

* Abs Wheel. One of my favorite exercises. This workout will make your core shiver. You can kneel on your knees, then move ahead on your Abs Wheel. If you're strong enough, you can elevate your legs and your toes becoming the only contact you have

with the ground. Perform 15 reps, then increase to 20 reps.

* Arms high, partial sit-up. Like the crunch lie down on your back with your heels flat to the floor with your knees wide and then raise your arms. Now , raise your upper body in a similar way as the crunch.

* Dip/Leg Raises Combo. Take the dip bar, then bend down and dip one time with your legs extended towards the sky. As you ascend you should circle your legs before you two times clockwise and two times counterclockwise. Then, go back down the dip. Repetition 5 times gradually working until you are able to do 10 times.

* Plank. A climber's essential. Start in a Plank position and place the weight of your forearms and the toes with your shoulders spread wide. Keep in the plank position for straight backs for at least for a minute, and work your way up to three minutes. It is also possible to put an exercise ball on your hips, and then take it off when you get tired.

* Side Plank. Another climber is essential for the your core muscles. Relax on your side with your weight resting on your forearms or using your hands, raise the other hand straight upwards. Maintain your body in a straight line and prevent your hips from sinking. Start with one minute, gradually increasing to 2 minutes per side.

* Russian Twist of the Medicine Ball. You should sit down with your legs bent and your feet lying flat on the ground. Place a 20-pound medicine in your hands. Rotate you upper body to the side. Do 20 repetitions.

* Hanging Leg Raises. Use a pull-up bar to hang and stretch your legs towards you. Perform 20 repetitions.

*TRX Snaps. The feet are placed in 2 TRX straps couple of inches higher than the floor. Relax your body and then rest your arms upon your arms. Now , move your body and bring your knees up to your chest. Do 20 quick repetitions.

*Jack Knives. Like we said earlier, lay on your back, flat on your stomach and extend your arms forwards and raise your legs and arms up at the same time. Make sure you are touching your ankles with your arms out and remain in a well-controlled, steady posture.

Sunday

Sunday is considered to be a "fun time". It should be an "wildcard" morning, based on your mood. If you are feeling that your body is in need of rest, follow your body's call. If you're feeling like being active, working with the outside of your boulders or running along the shore, or playing with your own American Ninja Obstacles in your backyard, do it. If you're feeling energetic enough to exercise, go to the gym and perform the "non-traditional" exercise. This means that you'll work on muscle groups that you do not focus on as often, like the your chest (doing the pushups Dumbbell Bench Press, Cable Flies, Incline, Decline) and shoulders (shoulder pressups and handstand squats against the wall dumbbell front raise, as well as side lift) or legs (military press deadlifts, squats and squats with different leg and foot position).

It is recommended to do pull-ups every day. If you spot the bar, leap on it and complete several repetitions. As I mentioned earlier I would highly suggest that purchasing a hang-board which you can put up on top of the door frame. It will allow you to do regular pull-ups using a variety of hand positions, and build your fingers and your core. The hang board is usually equipped with a variety of great workout suggestions. Make sure you get warm to prevent injuries to the tendon. If you do are able to train with real American Ninja Obstacles Train with them as often as you can to make sure you are comfortable with the way they operate.

Chapter 23: Surviving the toughest obstacles

Warning: Warm your body prior to exercising. Begin with a ten-minute light run, cycle or walk. Do a thorough stretch of your muscles particularly those which will be utilized (actively as well as passively) during your workout. It should take between 20 and 30 minutes to warm up , and be careful not to get injured. Injuries can delay you for several months, and may end your chances of competing in the competition.

Each Season of American Ninja Warrior alters the obstacles to a certain degree in an effort create a more thrilling for viewers. But, in the end, the obstacles remain the same that are focused on arm and balance, finger strength, endurance in anaerobic conditions and , of course, core strength.

Below are some difficult obstacles, as well as suggestions on how to construct these obstacles to increase your the strength and confidence. Although these obstacles won't be utilized in the current course however, they'll improve your skills, and could be applied to different obstaclesthat require similar strength and endurance.

Salmon Ladder

The Salmon Ladder has been on since the start of the show and is the most-feared obstacle in Sasuke as well as American Ninja Warrior, taking competitors out with a dozen. This Salmon Ladder evolved from a one-sided ladder , then double-sided ladders and, most recently, a swap salmon ladder which is actually a series of double salmon ladders making competitors switch directions numerous times. To conquer this challenge it requires more than just physical power. In contrast to other bridges, such as the Ultimate Cliffhanger or the Unstable Bridge the Salmon Ladder is highly technical and is a source of respect, because of numerous people who appear strong not achieving the ladder. To overcome the fear of the unknown and master the correct technique, I suggest that you construct an adirondack ladder. It can be easily and swiftly completed:

Two sturdy beams (or four for a double salmon ladder) and anchor them to the ground about 4 feet from each other. If you are able to locate two trees that are spaced approximately four feet apart it is also possible to use the beams.

* Purchase high-quality nails that are thick and strong in Home Depot and hammer them into the tree/beams at an angle of 35 degrees and then let them hang out about 3 inches.

Repeat the steps above climbing the trees/beams and spacing the rungs twelve inches between each until you are 12 feet tall.

* Finally, purchase a strong wooden bar, wooden bar, or an aluminum bar, that can be able to support your weight while suspended from the bar.

The obstacle you have in mind when you to train in your backyard will reduce the mental stigma associated with this obstacle. For the Salmon ladder, it is crucial to concentrate upon your core, and utilize the momentum. The Salmon ladder is basically similar movements to the exercise on campus that we discussed earlier. It is essential to strengthen your core and utilize the momentum of your legs. As you lift off, ensure you are pulling the bar straight at a similar force for each arm. Repeat the exercise several times a week to increase muscle memory.

Unstable Bridge

It is known as the Unstable Bridge, while looking like an easy obstacle that is easily overcome with solid upper body strength , keeps beating out competitors after competitors like Youuji Urushihara (Grand Champion) and Drew Dreschel (3 time American Ninja Warrior finalist). To conquer this challenge, you must develop the strength in the upper body as well as grip strength and core strength in order to successfully complete the gap leap. The thing that makes this challenge so difficult is that it is a bit late in the stage. At the point you reach the Unstable Bridge, your arms are pumping off to the ladder of salmon. The main skill apart of the evident upper arms strength, is the power of momentum. If you're imaginative, you can construct an own Unstable Bridge, hanging from an 8-oot support beam.

* You can construct two bridges using 2x4s or strong plywood and attach them

to the beam supporting. You can drill four holes on each corner, and then weave four ropes across the bridge before securing them by knots on the opposite side.

* In the second bridge, thread two ropes in the holes at the center and then secure them using knots on the opposite side of the hole.

These are the dimensions that follow:

* The length of the bridge is 4 feet

* Bridge Width is 1.5 feet

* Bridge Thickness : 1.25 inches

The gap between bridges of 1 foot

* The support beam must be at minimum 9 feet long

The most crucial tip to overcome this challenge is to hold your arms at an angle of 90 degrees. Don't allow your arms to hang down or move straight, because this makes it much more difficult to keep your balance while walking across the bridge.

Jumping Spider

The Jumping Spider been a difficult obstacle that is able to eliminate the most skilled competitors. Similar to similar to Salmon Ladder, you have to overcome your mental block first . Then, be aware that the obstacle its own isn't too difficult. Instead of strength, you will require an abundance of energy and concentration. You should aim forward and up around a 45-55 degree angle. Once you've made contact, pull your legs and arms away and stop the forward motion. It is possible to test the sudden motion between door frames. If you own an Parkour running facility close to you, I suggest switching up your training routines by doing periodic Parkour exercise and obstacle training. This will not only boost your confidence and remove the "fear" of both mental and physical obstacles, it will you will also increase your the body's control, thereby increasing endurance, strength and flexibility, as well as agility, balance as well as explosive force. If there isn't the facilities of a Parkour facility in your area simply go outside and utilize natural or constructed obstacles during your training. Although you might consider that your local area isn't equipped with sufficient obstacles entire concept behind Parkour is to make use of whatever obstacles you encounter. A simple wall or railing could make a great tool for training.

Cliffhanger

The most hated obstacle in American Ninja Warrior. This challenge requires a strong fingers and upper body strength. If you're doing your exercises, particularly on campus, you can overcome this obstacle in the blink of an eye. What makes it difficult is that once you get to this point, you're already pumped by the previous hurdles. Get your endurance up at the rock climbing gym by performing your drills and traverses on your 4x4s. Begin by completing at least half an hour of climbing without touching the ground.

A brief note on how to conquer difficulties by utilizing Parkour

Parkour, sometimes known as Freerunning is becoming quite popular in the last few years. Parkour helps the body as well as your mind how to over come obstacles at a speed and with efficiency which requires flexibility and creativity as well as a strategies. To be able to overcome any obstacle (and not be injured!) the parkour-loving athletes also referred to as traceurs or traceuses, learn to view the world in a different manner by using actions such as running, vaulting and climbing, swinging and balancing, to move through, over and over obstacles. If you're fortunate enough to have an Parkour running facility close to you, I would suggest switching up your training routine by adding occasionally Parkour exercise and training. It will not only boost your confidence and allow you to overcome the fear of failure, set goals and think critically to conquer physical and mental obstacles, but it will also help improve the body's control and increase strength and endurance, as well as agility, balance, flexibility and explosive force. If there isn't an Parkour gym in your neighborhood simply go outside and make use of natural or artificial obstacles during your training. Although you might believe that your location doesn't have many obstacles to overcome, remember that the main purpose of Parkour is to make use of whatever obstacles you encounter. A simple wall or railing could make a great tool for training.

Chapter 24: Ninja Nutrition

Disclaimer This diet advice or meal programs are just suggestions to follow to build strength and energy. The below food suggestions have worked for me personally and for many other athletes as can be seen on websites, such as www.livestrong.com or www.fitnessmagazine.com as well as books written by pro athletes such as "All-Pro Diet" by Tony Gonzalez.

In order to be able to prepare effectively for to be prepared for American Ninja Warrior competition you should make sure the body in good fitness. Training without the proper fuel won't get you far. Like I said I would suggest you begin your training at least a year prior to the start of your test-outs. You will be expected to work out frequently and hard, which will require you to exercise with a lot of determination and enthusiasm. Keep in mind, "You are what you take in!" First and foremost eliminate any processed food items, like the ones you love like McDonalds cheeseburger soda, as well as French fries. I would generally suggest you prepare your own meals to know the ingredients that are employed. The majority of restaurants use harmful Canola Oil, which you should substitute by Coconut and Avocado Oil. It is vital to keep a healthy diet that includes protein, carbohydrates and fiber.

The Paleo Diet

A Paleo diet can be described as the best diet for athletes who compete since it's the only diet that integrates your genes to allow you to remain strong, lean and active. Recent studies in biology, biochemistry and ophthalmology, among many other fields has revealed that a diet based on processed foods and trans fats, and sugar is the most significant cause of degenerative illnesses such as diabetes, cancer, obesity heart disease, cancer, and many more diseases, and that's not even mentioning the lack of energy levels and a lack of performance as a result.

In essence In a nutshell Paleo diet is comprised of fibrous foods like fruits and vegetables that replenish your body with antioxidants as well as enzymes and minerals and protein food items that guarantee the health of your muscles and overall energy. Without getting too involved in details of the diet, I'll give you an easy-to-follow weekly menu plan. You can follow this plan for two weeks and notice the improvement in your level of energy, overall wellbeing and your body's overall slimness.

Here's a quick outline on the Paleo Diet "eat" and "don't take a break from eating" list.

Eat

Grass-fed meats. Enjoy all types of meats and avoid high-fat cuts. I suggest turkey, poultry and pork, as well as bison, beef and duck.

Fish/seafood. Seafood tends to be extremely thin. Try eating salmon, bass trout, red snapper tuna, halibut, halibut as well as lobster, shrimp, and shrimp.

Fresh fruits. Fruits with a low amount of sugar are beneficial because they can increase your energy levels and give you a feeling of being refreshed and refreshed. The most popular are citrus, lime, lemon apple, pear squash, pumpkin and zucchini. They also include tomato cucumber, bell pepper and avocado.

Fresh vegetables. Water chestnuts are a good choice parsley, jicama shallots, scallions, fennel leek, garlic turnip, asparagus watercress, radishes celery, bok-choy as well as green beans alfalfa, artichokes, alfalfa spro sauerkraut Brussels sprouts as well as cauliflower, onions, mushrooms cabbage, chard, broccoli, kale as well as collard greens.

Starchy vegetables. I love adding them into my diet because they bring me a more full feeling, without feeling tired. Take a bite of the butternut squash, yams beets, and sweet potato.

Eggs. I love eggs. They are a great source of protein and taste delicious. Try different varieties like duck, chicken Quil, ostrich, and quail.

Nuts. These are excellent snacks to have during workouts. Consume many cashews, almonds hazelnuts and brazil nuts walnuts, pecans, and walnuts.

Seeds. Seeds can be incorporated into any dish to give you an extra energy boost. The most recommended seeds include the sunflower seeds and pumpkin seeds flax seeds, and chia seeds.

Healthy oils. Your body requires fats that is healthy fat. Healthy fats aid in the conversion of glucose into energy for your body to remain active and vibrant. Cook your food with avocado and coconut oil and olive oil. You can also use walnut oil, olive oil, and pumpkin seed oil for the meals (remember not to cook olive oil) as well as add fish oil to curries you love.

Seasonings, Condiments and herbs. Chili, Hot Sauce horseradish, tapenade, and mustard are the best selections. Avoid packaged versions as much as possible. Be sure to check if the product contains lots of soy or sugar. Choose products with less sodium instead.

DO NOT EAT

Fattier meats like hot spam, dogs or other poor quality cuts

Cereal grains

Legumes include lentils, beans, peas Tofu, soybeans peanuts, peanut butter miso, and so on.)

Dairy

Artificial sweeteners and refined sugar

Potatoes

Processed food products

Foods that are salty or overly salted

Refined vegetable oils

Junk food, candy or processed foods

Fruit Juices

Alcohol

Sodas

Sample Meal Plans

I've provided some meal plans that I have sampled that offer simple and quick ways of cooking delicious meals that allow your body to stay active all daylong. You are at ease to experiment and experiment with variations you'd like, using the "eat/don't consume" guide to use as a source of. Naturally, there are hundreds of delicious recipes to follow eating the Paleo diet. These recipes that I have personally tried and tested are just a start for you to try. For me, it's essential to cook a delicious dinner without having to stand at the stove for long. I also enjoy cooking large portions, which gives me delicious leftover meals later in the day.

Breakfast

California Omelet

* 4-5 cage-free eggs

* 1 tsp avocado oil

* 1 Onion cut into pieces

* 1 cup spinach, chopped

* 1 teaspoon fresh basil

* 1 handful of cocktail tomatoes, cut in half

* 1 Avocado, cut into slices

* 2 bacon strips (optional)

Salt as well as Pepper

Break eggs into bowls add salt and pepper, and mix until they are well blended. Cook onions in a skillet until translucent. Mix egg mixture in and cook for about a few minutes. Then add tomatoes, spinach and basil, and then spread them over the egg mixture. Then flip one side on top of the other side and cook until the egg mixture is no longer liquid. Serving alongside Avocados as a side along with your preferred hot sauce.

Power Shake

One small beet in red or cut a large one in half

* 1 carrot

2. Leaves of Kale

* 1 Celery

* One thumb Ginger

* 1 Orange

* 1 Apple

* 1 Banana

* 1tsp Avocado Oil or Coconut Oil

Peel and chop ingredients in blender. Add two to three cups oil and water, and blend for one minute until the ingredients are all pureed. Serving size. 4 cups. Consume right away.

Note: This recipe will ensure that you'll be filled with minerals and vitamins for the next day. I suggest using natural fruits and veggies. For more details on the different types of juices look up the appendix that contains my book recommendations.

Carrot along with Zucchini Scramble

* 4-5 cage-free eggs

* 1 carrot cut into pieces, preferring to be processed in food processor

* 1 Zucchini chopped, preferred in food processor

1 Tbsp Coconut Oil

* Salt, and Pepper

In a pan, heat oil Add zucchini and carrots and fry for one minute, while stirring. Add eggs as well as salt and pepper according to your preference and stir often until eggs are set.

Coconut Flour Pancakes

* 3 Tbsp Coconut Flour

* 3 Eggs

2TBSp unsweetened apple sauce

* 3-4 tbsp Coconut Milk

1 Tbsp Coconut Oil

* 1/4 teaspoon Baking Soda

* 1-2 Tbsp Coconut Sugar

* 1/4 tsp Organic Apple Cider Vinegar

Mix egg and flour until you get an easy-to-mix paste. Add apple sauce as well as coconut sugar and coconut milk mixing until the mixture is smooth. Just before the pancakes are cooked you can add baking soda. In a pan, heat oil and then add small portions of pancake batter and cook until golden brown the pancakes on both sides. Serve by serving it with fruit juice and honey or Strawberry sauce (1 cup strawberries, 2 tablespoons coconut cream and 1 tablespoon honey, mixed).

Lunch

Ceviche

* 1 lbs fresh , uncooked fish fillet

* 5 limes

* 4 cloves garlic

* 1 Tbsp fresh cilantro

* 1 jalapeno chili

1. 1 tiny red onion chopped

* 8 large romaine lettuce leaves

* 1 Avocado, diced

* 1 tomato diced

* Salt, and Pepper

* Hot Sauce

Cube the fish and place it in a glass bowl. Juice limes in food processor. Add cilantro, garlic and seeded jalapeno. Chop into fine pieces. Mix with fish and add onions. Let it marinate overnight. Prior to eating, you can remove most lime juice, leaving the fish in a moist state. Add the salt as well as pepper. The recipe can be doubled to take meals for two days. The lime is an organic preservative to the fish.

Chicken Salad

* 1 lb organic chicken

1/4 cup red bell pepper diced

* One artichoke heart chopped and cooked

* 2 scallions, thinly cut* 2 scallions, thinly sliced

* 1 tbsp fresh parsley, minced

* 1/3 cup mayonnaise (optional Mix it with 1 tbsp lemon , one clove of garlic)

* 1 Tbsp Coconut Oil

* 1 Avocado

In a pan, heat oil and add the chicken. Season lightly by adding salt and black pepper. After chicken is cooked to your liking, take it off the heat and mix with the other ingredients in the bowl. Mix well, and serve with a freshly cut Avocado as a side.

Oven roasted vegetable

* 1 Zucchini Cut into smaller pieces

* 1 yellow squash

* 1 red bell pepper removed and cut into tiny pieces

* 1 lb fresh green asparagus, cut in smaller pieces

* 1 onion red

* Salt, and Pepper

* 2 Tbsp Coconut Oil

The oven should be heated to 450F. Mix all vegetables into the roasting pan. Add salt, oil, and pepper, and mix thoroughly. Spread the vegetables out. Roast for 30 minutes until golden brown. You can store the leftovers in the refrigerator and take them cold to eat in the future.

Dinner

Chicken Curry

* 6 boneless thighs of chicken (organic when is possible)

* 1 onion chopped

1. 1 cup of coconut milk, or puree pumpkin (using canned purée is acceptable)

* 2 medium zucchinis, sliced

* 2 cups crimini mushrooms

* 1/2 teaspoon Turmeric powder

* 1/2 tsp Paprika powder

* 1 tsp red pepperflakes

* 1 teaspoon Cumin

* 2 Tbsp Coconut Oil

Cook the oil in a pan and add onions and cook until they are browned. Add the spices to the onions and stir for about a minute until they are fragrant. Add the chicken and cook until the chicken is cooked through and sides turn white. Then add the coconut milk or pumpkin puree along with a tiny amount of water. Stir thoroughly. Cover the curry and let it simmer until it has a the flavor. After 10 minutes, add the zucchinis as well as mushrooms. Cook for 5 minutes more and Serve with freshly chopped cilantro as well as a splash in coconut cream.

I like to make a big portion to heat up over the next two days. The curries will get better when they are stored in your refrigerator.

Steak and sweet Potatoes

* 1 steak cut you like (Sirloin or New York are my favorites)

* Salt, pepper and salt

* 2 tsp Avocado Oil

* 1 lbs sweet potatoes

Cut sweet potatoes in half. Peel them and cut them in half. Be sure that the pieces of potato aren't too large. Set your oven at 350F, and bake the potatoes for at least an one hour. When they're done, you'll be able to tell when they're soft and fluffy and sweet. In the meantime, sprinkle your the steak liberally with salt and black pepper, then sprinkle it with avocado oil. Ten minutes prior to when the potatoes are cooked cook the oil in an iron skillet . Then cook your steak. You can then serve according to your preference. I like medium-rare so I let the steak rest for 1 to 2 minutes each side. Add a slice of onion to the skillet if you want to add some flavor. A serving of avocado as a side dish is delicious.

Beef Chili

* 2 pounds ground beef

* 1 red and green bell pepper

* 1 large onion, diced

* 5 cloves of garlic that are medium in size

* 2 tbsp Avocado Oil

* 2 fresh tomatoes, diced

* 1 Jalapeno de-seeded, cut into smaller pieces

* 3 Tbsp Cumin powder

* 2 tbsp Chili powder

The pan is heated and you can add onions. Add ground beef, and sprinkle with the salt as well as pepper. Once the beef is nearly cooked, Add Cumin as well as Chili powders. Stir thoroughly. Add other ingredients and then add the drinking water until it covers all ingredients. Allow the chili to simmer for about an hour, stirring frequently.

Snacks

* Nuts. You can buy a complete bag of mixed, unsalted nuts at Sprouts, and mix these with raisins and raisins or.

* Banana Bread. I bake Paleo banana bread every week and consume it when I am hungry.

* Avocadoes. Avocados are delicious when eaten along with organic Ryvita. A minimum of 1/3 avocado spread on organic rye toast can provide you with a

lot of great since it's tasty and high in fiber.

* A potent yet light smoothie that is light but powerful. Mixing bananas blueberries, bananas, and honey is a potent smoothie , particularly after drinking a mixture of raw greens, nut butter protein powder, the fruit of your choice. A healthy smoothie can rev up your mood and boost your energy regardless of what time of morning it's. Blended berries frozen and almond milk can help.

* Dry fruits and whole nuts. It's your health-conscious version of trail mix or granola and is one of those foods you'd love eating.

* Bananas. Bananas contain the right amount of carbs sugar fiber, potassium, and sugar making them the ideal snack to eat before a workout or a game. Be sure to have some to you at all times.

*Carrots for Baby Children/Carrot Sticks. Carrot sticks for babies may be a little sweet but they don't contain lots of sugar. They actually contain plenty of fiber to sustain your body and help you stay active. Take them along with hummus, or a natural nut butter, and you're good to go!

Chapter 25: Finding the Job

This is perhaps the toughest aspect of being a stuntman especially when you're getting started in the industry. Nobody is aware of who you are or what you're capable of doing.

In the case of an actor you'd have to go on auditions. There may be auditions for stunt performers, regardless of whether they're for film, television, or live performances. If you're in that situation, here are some important points to be aware of...

There's a lot tension in a stunt audition when you watch other performers cowboy it up. There is a temptation to go that are beyond your capabilities. Don't. Not only could you be seriously injured, but if you do not succeed, you'll be a failure before the whole community. The word spreads. There's no pressure here. Take what you can.

The only exception could be Zoe Bell, who was auditioning for Quentin Tarantino's "Kill Bill." The actress kept falling down as she tried a trick with an impromptu tramp. But she kept getting up. This is what impressed Tarantino and earned her the role (watch Double Dare).

I've attended a few auditions where participants have made incredibly poor choices. I've seen people hurt their ankle while jumping on a trampoline. They've also seen them stab or kick their opponent in an altercation, fall thirty feet into the air in a bid to slip down the rope, then hit the water with a sideways kick from fifty feet and then fall on their heads performing a tumbling sequence due to the fact that they had having a floor made of springs instead of carpet.

In that vein I attended an audition in martial arts, where they wanted to test some moves in real time. Without thinking, I did the heel spin quickly that I've tried a million times, and I completely didn't realize that I was in tennis footwear on carpet. I nearly snapped the knee.

But I did get an interview... Here's what you need to know: If you show up for an audition for a fight the judges will match you up with a stranger who might not have expertise or may try to take you down. You'll have just ten minutes to learn an act that could make you squirm. Instead, bring your partner to fight with you over something has been working for many months. Casting won't be able to tell what's going on and will surprise them!

Be nice to everyone you meet at an audition. You never know who will be watching. When I help select the fighters for a show, I usually meet up with the actors. Most of them have no clue who I am, and I can see the person they are. I am able to observe their attitudes. It's hilarious when someone with a snarky self-centered attitude walks to the office and spots me sitting with Director of Casting. But they won't receive the job.

However, auditioning is only one aspect of getting work in the field of stunts. This is also an apprenticeship. It's about making yourself known as a professional. It can be an extended process before people recognize your name and the things you accomplish.

Start by experimenting with student films, freebies or non-union-sponsored shows. Contrary to what many believe it is a valuable aspect in the learning process. In addition to the practical knowledge The people who you meet could later become your friends who are stunt experts director, coordinators, or coordinators.

Patience. It could take years to perfect your abilities, make the appropriate connections, and build an image as a professional stunt performer. The first job isn't easy, particularly when stunt coordinators tend to select the same performers repeatedly and over. At first, I thought it was an indication of nepotism however, I came to realize that it was about trust.

If you're at an edge in a structure getting ready to leap and fall, you need to be sure that the person who controls that airbag is aware of the risks. You're entrusting them with your life. That type of trust isn't something you can see on a job or demo reel.

This is why you must collaborate. This is why that you should learn from professionals in the field. Your colleagues should trust that you are assured that you'll do the job correctly, and to not end up killing anyone. This is logical.

Working with professionals provides you with the chance to meet people and get noticed. Every stuntman has a story to tell of getting in the correct spot at the right moment. Attending a training session with professionals in stunts is the best place to be.

A few years ago, I took my friend to a workout for stunts. He had a little fight training however, he had never attempted high falls or used an improvised tramp in his entire life. The next day an stunt coordinator turned up and picked a group of random men, including him, to create a major Clint Eastwood film for two months. The right location at the right time.

Sometimes, they might be seeking to duplicate a certain actor or body type, and you may just be perfect for the job. Quentin Tarantino found Zoe Bell during a stunt training during her first week in LA and instantly hired her to play Uma Thurman for Kill Bill.

I was first offered an SAG job while I was training for an exercise with swords as a stunt manager spotted that I was an ideal match with David Hasselhoff.

Perhaps you have a special talent. My wife is proficient at double whips , not something women are able to do. A stunt coordinator saw her working out at a fitness class and suggested her to a television show that required her exact abilities. In addition to bringing her to be a part of the SAG weekly, they also requested casting for an actress who was similar to her.

Nearly every stuntman has an account like this. While these opportunities do occur in LA however, they are extremely scarce. If you're trying to find jobs that you can count on it is essential to "hustle."

"Hustling" is how most indie stunt performers find work. You discover which film is shooting and arrive with the resume and headshot over to the director of the scene.

To locate the location the film's location actors will inquire one another (word from mouth) or travel to typical locations for filming, such as downtown LA. They also get tips online from the Hollywood Reporter or sites like OnLocationVacation.com. Learn about the shooting locations and who's coordinating the shoot.

There are also breakdown services, such as "Stunt Contact" and "Stunt Listing Breakdown" which (for cost) can provide you with regularly scheduled breakdowns for action movies and shoot dates, production details and the details of the respective coordinators for stunts, as well as contact information to submit your resume.

The most difficult aspect of hustling is to get the stunt coordinator's attention on the set. I suggest that you meet with a stunt performer (preferably one who is able to present you) and wait for the right time. It is usually about lunchtime or 6 hours after the call time (noon for the majority of shoots).

A few stunt actors prefer showing on time at the beginning of the shoot day, which is often very late (5-6am). It's all about timing and there are a few stories of stunt performers being hired right away (so it's a good idea to pack your gear in your vehicle). When I first got employed as a coordinator, I was hired by the man to work as a stunt-related utility.

Be aware that you shouldn't try to speak to the same person all the time. The usual rule of thumb is every month, once or twice.

Be open to unconventional ways of hustling. If you've got your resume or card with your person, any time could result in your next job.

The other day at AFM (the American Film Market) I spotted the poster for a movie named Sinbad that was currently in preproduction. I delivered a headshot as well as a resume at the office of the production and within three weeks I was flying for Jordan for the role of the combat coordinator.

Be aware that there's an issue as excessive hustle and it can cause annoyance with you (friends and family members) If you only push everybody. I've witnessed this work against stunt performers who have lost jobs due to it. Be sure to keep a steady pace.

Personally, I've never been enthusiastic about hustling. I am a firm believer in making my own work and therefore I'm not in a waiting room for my phone to start to ring (see my previous chapter).

Again, my most important advice is to learn with those who are working in the field. My second recommendation is to meet people. The old adage "it's whom you're with" is completely true. Stunt performers form a close-knit group, and frequently employ someone they know better than an individual with more experience.

There are many events that are industry-related like the Stunt Softball League Bowling in stunts, Xmas at the Stuntmen's Association and The Stunt Emmys , World Stunt Awards, Dragonfest and Wally Crowder's "hustle night" that can help keep people in mind what you look like. Don't forget to attend an opportunity to attend a party at Morgan's home.

Don't forget to use social media. Look on Facebook for groups such as The Stunt People's Availability Checklist as well as any other groups for stunts that you might discover. It's free to join groups and you'll don't know what you might find when you involved which is why you should go wild. Be careful not to fall into that Facebook rabbit hole, or you'll end up spending longer on your laptop than in the studio.

Then, you can find other people to work with you. Visit the section I have of "Agencies" and sign up with online services such as Actors Access and Backstage.

Be honest about your capabilities! "Fake it till you create it" is a good idea as a stage act, but with stunts, it could be fatal. It is tempting to work for a company which requires skills that you do not possess. Don't. Even a small mistake made wrong could have severe consequences - and If not for you, then another person. In the end lying about your capabilities could end your professional career.

The same as securing the job, it isn't being hired. It is easy to get yourself into a tizzy thinking about why they hired an employee other than you, and not get an answer. It's okay to let it slide.

Everybody living in LA will have a personal story to tell about an opportunity missed. I'd been trying to join the Highlander TV series for years and had finally gave up. I was on set for the other series when I received an unknown call from an area code . I chose to respond at work. I came home at night and checked the messages and found "This call is from an office from the Highlander producer's office. Please contact us whenever you can. We'd love to have you as a guest on the next episode. ..."

Conclusion

Thank you so much for purchasing this book!

I hope that this book was helpful in getting you familiar with and be inspired through the sport of parkour as well as freerunning.

Next step, you must get out to the world and continue training. Parkour and freerunning aren't races, and it's best to view them as life-styles. Take your own route, and have fun along the way.

Thanks for your kind words and best wishes!

www.ingramcontent.com/pod-product-compliance
Lightning Source LLC
Chambersburg PA
CBHW050023130526
44590CB00042B/1869